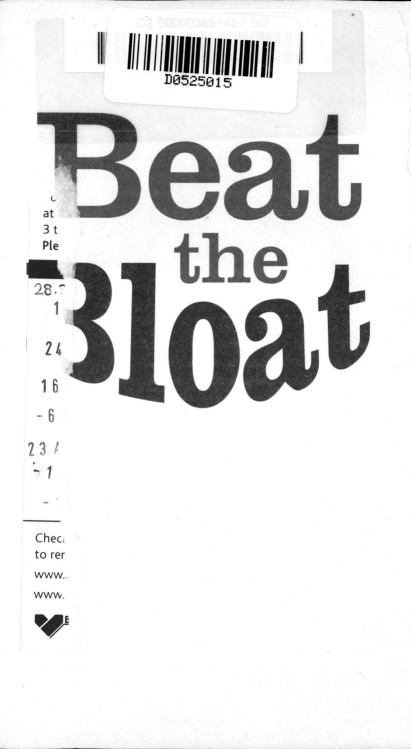

Beat
the
Bloat

hamlyn

Beat the Bloat

Lose weight, feel great!

Helen Foster
Recipes by Louise Blair

An Hachette Livre UK Company

First published in Great Britain in 2008 by
Hamlyn, a division of Octopus Publishing Group Ltd
2-4 Heron Quays, London E14 4JP
www.octopusbooks.co.uk

ISBN 978-0-600-61681-8

A CIP catalogue record for this book is available from the British Library

Printed and bound in Great Britain by Mackays of Chatham

10 9 8 7 6 5 4 3 2 1

Both metric and imperial measurements are given for the recipes. Use one set of measures
only, not a mixture of both.

Ovens should be preheated to the specified temperature. If using a fan-assisted oven,
follow the manufacturer's instructions for adjusting the time and temperature. Grills
should also be preheated.

This book includes dishes made with nuts and nut derivatives. It is advisable for those with
known allergic reactions to nuts and nut derivatives and those who may be potentially
vulnerable to these allergies, such as pregnant and nursing mothers, invalids, the elderly,
babies and children, to avoid dishes made with nuts and nut oils. It is also prudent to check
the labels of prepared ingredients for the possible inclusion of nut derivatives.

The Department of Health advises that eggs should not be consumed raw. It is prudent for
more vulnerable people such as pregnant and nursing mothers, invalids, the elderly, babies
and young children to avoid uncooked or lightly cooked dishes made with eggs.

This book should not be considered a replacement for professional medical treatment;
a physician should be consulted on all matters relating to health. While the advice and
information in this book are believed to be accurate, neither the author nor the publisher
can accept any legal responsibility for any illness sustained while following the advice
in this book.

Contents

Introduction

What is bloat?

You wake up in the morning feeling slim and trim, but by mid-afternoon everything changes. Your waistband feels tight and you may need to loosen your belt a notch. From the side, you look 'pregnant' and you may also be suffering side-effects such as stomach cramps or gassy episodes. That's bloat – one type of it anyway. The other type is the feeling of puffiness you get on hot days or, for women, around the time of your period, when it's not just your tummy that's swollen but your face, fingers and ankles too. Whichever type you suffer it's not fun, and it's often enough to trigger some seriously drastic diet plans to beat it.

False fat

The problem is that, while we might feel as if we need to slim when it hits us, bloat is not fat. We gain fat when excess calories cause the tiny little fat cells around our middles to expand in size – when this occurs, the fat stays put until you deprive your body of extra calories, usually through a diet or exercise plan, meaning that your body must dip into those fat cells for extra fuel. Bloat, however, is a temporary sensation that merely makes you feel as if you've gained weight for a few hours, or days, at a time. That might sound

'Over four million women in the UK sought help for bloat-related issues in 2006 alone.'

preferable to actual weight gain but, while you can adapt and disguise true fat while you work on losing it, bloat – or false fat, as it is also known – can hit without warning, causing you to go up one or even two clothing sizes around your middle in a matter of hours, often accompanied by a dose of discomfort or outright pain. With bloat, you can start the day at 63 kg (140 lb/10 stone) and end up looking (and potentially weighing) 70 kg (154 lb/11 stone). An outfit you felt fabulous in at 9 am can be tight and unflattering by 3 pm. While bloat might only be temporary, it will sap your confidence as fast as any extra true additions on the scales when it does hit.

And it does. According to market research group IPSOS Mori in the UK, over four million women sought help from their doctor or pharmacist for bloat-related issues in the year of 2006 alone – and you can bet that millions more suffered in silence. But bloat is not solely a feminist issue. Modern life is making men more bloat-prone too: our low-nutrient diets, hurried, stressful lives and even the fact that we are living longer are making both genders more prone to the false fat epidemic. Know what causes your problem, though, and you can determine how to beat it – for good.

Can you beat the bloat and lose weight too?

✣ Yes, the plans in this book aim primarily to fight the triggers behind bloat, but because many people who suffer bloat would also like to lose weight the plans are designed to make that happen too. Each of them contains around 1,400 calories a day, which will lead to a weight loss of around half a kilo (1 lb) a week for women, and slightly more for men, which is safe and sustainable. If you don't want to lose weight, you'll need to add 400–800 more calories each day by increasing portion sizes and/or adding at least one more snack.

What causes bloat?

Bloat is caused by two main biological factors – the production of too much gas, or the retention of too much fluid. These produce either a swelling of the stomach or intestines, or a plumping of the tissues of the body, causing the 'suddenly fat' sensation. The complicated thing about bloat, however, is that these two primary causes can have a number of triggers. The most common triggers are described below.

Digestive disorders

Normally food passes through the digestive system fairly rapidly – in fact within as little as five hours of eating it, an item you've consumed can be processed and in the large intestine waiting to be excreted within 12–24 hours. However, if problems with your digestive system slow down this process, food will ferment in the stomach or intestines and gas will form. These problems can include intolerance to common foods, a lack of the digestive enzymes that help break down food in the stomach, or lowered levels of the good bacteria that tackle it in the intestines – but they all cause abdominal swelling and the bloat that comes with it.

Hormonal changes

A very common cause of bloat in women. The menstrual cycle is controlled by fluctuations in the hormones oestrogen and progesterone occurring throughout the month. Both of these can be linked to fluid retention, but with premenstrual syndrome (PMS) the hormone progesterone is the most commonly discussed trigger. One of the many jobs of this hormone is to stimulate kidney function and fluid excretion in the body; just prior to your period progesterone levels fall and these functions slow up, meaning that you physically excrete less fluid each day, and the fluid that is retained leaks from inside the cells through the capillary walls to the spaces around them, causing puffiness.

Dietary factors

Modern diets are made to bloat us. Many of us skip meals or eat too quickly, both of which can lead to gas creation in the stomach and intestine. We're also eating diets that increase both fluid- and air-related gas in the system by depriving us of some vital nutrients, and overloading our system with some less essential ones such as sodium. Finally, there are food intolerances – up to 90 per cent of some populations suffer these to some degree – and bloat is one of the primary symptoms.

Lymphatic issues

Imagine the lymph system of your body as a series of canals, pushing fluid around your system to areas such as the armpits, kidneys and bowels where it can be excreted in sweat, urine and faeces. If those canals stagnate, nothing goes anywhere and fluid pools in the body, causing bloat. One of the biggest factors that controls lymph movement is movement of the muscles – meaning exercise; in a world where, according to the British Chiropractic Association, nearly a third of us sit for ten hours a day, and 29 per cent of us exercise only once a month or less, it's clear to see why that system is also breaking down.

‘ Bloat is caused either by the production of too much gas or the retention of too much fluid. ,

With all these causes of bloat, clearly there is no one solution to the problem, which is why the first step in beating your bloat is learning which particular trigger(s) is causing yours. The quiz on pages 12–15 is the simplest way to do just that.

What's your problem?

Take a look at these 30 questions and tick any to which you answer yes. Now note the letter next to each of the ones you have ticked, and count up how many of each letter apply to you. The one that appears most for you is your primary bloat trigger and determines which plan you should be following in the rest of this book.

1   Do you suffer from runny nose, headaches, stomach upsets, mood swings, fatigue, hayfever, eczema or other odd health issues along with your bloating? (I)
2   Look at your tongue. Does it have indent marks down the side or a line down the middle? (D)
3   Have your symptoms got worse with age – particularly if you're over 40? (D)
4   Do your fingers, ankles, knees or face puff up if it's hot or you've been standing around for a while? (F)
5   Do you find you really crave certain foods – not sweets, but things such as pizza, pasta, cheese or milk? (I)
6   Would you describe your life as busy, manic, hectic, out of control – or any similar phrase? (S)
7   If you gain 'real' weight, does it go on predominantly around your middle? (S)
8   Do you know, or suspect, that your bloat gets worse if you eat a specific food? (I)
9   Do you eat wheat-based foods at almost every meal? (I)
10 Do you have dark circles under your eyes even though you're not tired? (I)
11 Do you wake up with a flat tummy but find it swells throughout the day? (D, I, S)
12 For women, do your symptoms occur primarily before your period? (F)
13 Do you spend fewer than ten minutes over a meal? (D, S)

14 Do you sleep fewer than eight hours a night? (S)

15 Do you go more than 48 hours without passing a stool? (D)

16 Do you tend to sleep on your right side? (D)

17 Are you often thirsty? (F)

18 Do you find you burp or pass gas a lot? (D, I)

19 If you answered yes to question 18, can you link this to any specific food? (I)

20 Press your ankle with your finger for 30 seconds. Does the skin stay indented for five seconds or more? (F, I)

21 Do your bloat symptoms worsen when you're tired? (S)

22 Do you skip meals or regularly leave more than four hours between them? (D, S)

23 Do you have stomach cramps or loose bowels? (S, I)

24 If you answered yes to question 23, can you attribute these to specific meals? (I)

25 If you answered yes to question 23, do the problems occur predominantly when you're stressed? (S)

26 Is your urine dark yellow? (F)

27 Do you eat lots of ready meals, processed meats, tinned soups and/or breakfast cereals? (F)

28 Do you cook with salt or add it to your meals once they've been served? (F)

29 Do your symptoms vanish if you go on holiday? (S)

30 Do you drink fewer than eight 250 ml (8 fl oz) glasses of water a day? (F)

If you ticked mostly Is
It's likely that a food intolerance is to blame for your problems. The most common foods that trigger these are those containing wheat and dairy, so turn to page 20 where you'll find a plan that eliminates these two major culprits from your diet and should also eliminate bloat.

If you ticked mostly Ds
Digestive issues are behind your bloat. From page 66, you'll find a plan that aims to 'make over' your body from within by increasing levels of your digestive enzymes and the healthy bacteria that your system needs to thrive. You'll also learn that how you eat could be as important as what you're eating.

If you ticked mostly Fs
The biggest likely cause for your bloat symptoms is fluid retention, and this is far more likely to apply to women than to men. On page 112 you'll find the plan that aims to fight this by causing the excretion of excess fluid. Whether your problems occur only just before your period, or you suffer fluid retention all month, this plan will help.

If you ticked mostly Ss
Then you could be shocked to hear that your stressful life is likely to be the biggest factor behind your bloat. Turn to page 158 and you'll find a plan that aims to calm your mind – and your body – using a mix of dietary changes and psychological tips and tricks.

No clear trigger?

❋ It's possible that some people won't get a clear answer from this quiz, as two or even three letters might appear equally frequently. This can happen because the triggers that cause bloat can become linked – for example, a period of stress can trigger a food intolerance to manifest or disrupt your digestive enzymes; for women, if you're premenstrual you might be more stressed than normal, so think your problem is caused by your frazzled nerves when it's actually caused by your fluctuating hormones. If you currently have no clear answer to what might be potentially causing your bloat, choose one of the two solutions below.

Solution 1: First check your answers to questions 1, 2, 12, 20 and 29. These are very specific indicators for each of the bloat causes suggested. If you ticked yes to only one of those, that's the eating plan that will benefit you most – but also read the 'tip boxes' for your other potential triggers as they could help you break some other bloat-boosting habits that might otherwise derail your diet efforts.

Solution 2: If when you check questions 1, 2, 12, 20 and 29 you have ticked yes to one or more, then you probably have a couple of causes for your bloat. In this case, you can either choose to follow the plan you instinctively feel will give you the most benefit, or check which of the most-ticked letters appears first in this list – I, D, F, S. That's the order in which plans are likely to give the biggest benefits if your problems are more complex – but, again, read the 'tip boxes' for your other plans as well.

Your questions answered

With every organized diet plan there are always some questions. Some frequently asked ones are answered here.

If I don't like something on this diet, can I change ingredients?
Generally yes. There's no point giving anyone a diet plan they don't like to follow so you can swap like for like (one fish for another, or vegetables for salad). However, some ingredients in each plan are in there because of their specific health benefits, so do check the 'tip boxes' on each page to ensure that the ingredient you're completely avoiding isn't one that will do you the most good.

I work, so how is this diet going to fit into my life?
Almost every meal that's suggested as a lunchtime meal in the plans can be made before you get to work and taken in, or is available in most food shops and outlets. The meals on days 6–7 and 13–14 on each plan may require a little more preparation; this is because most people begin diet plans on a Monday, so it's assumed that these are weekend days. If they fall on your weekdays, though, it's no problem to swap the order of complete days around (but not individual meals – see next question).

Can I swap meals between days?
It's not recommended, since the days are designed to ensure you're getting a good mix of nutrients between the various meals.

I am vegetarian, so can I still follow these diets?
Yes. Every meal is either vegetarian or has a vegetarian option. The main recipes may sound meat-orientated in the diet plan description, but if you turn to the relevant page you will find a vegetarian alternative at the end of all of them.

I hate cooking, so do I really have to follow the recipes?

No. Whenever a recipe is suggested, there's a simple 'easy cook' alternative if you don't have the time or energy to cook on that day.

I don't want to lose weight, so would like to add the extra calories you suggested on page 9, but haven't a clue where to start. What do you suggest I do?

The easiest way to do it is to just add a selection of the following to the diets as needed (remembering to fit the rules of your plan):

- piece of fruit – 50 calories
- boiled egg – 90 calories
- slice of bread – 90 calories
- 25 g (1 oz) pasta/rice – 100 calories
- 125 g (4 oz) pot of natural yogurt – 100 calories
- a handful of nuts – 115 calories
- apple, topped with 2 teaspoons peanut butter – 170 calories
- 200 ml (7 fl oz) whole milk and 2 scoops whey protein powder – 200 calories
- 200 g (7 oz) potato – 260 calories

I know I suffer from bloat, but I think I also need to lose some weight. How can I tell?

The easiest way is to calculate your body mass index (BMI), which measures weight in relation to height. To do this, divide your weight in kilograms by your height in metres squared. If the figure you come up with is under 19.5, you are underweight and you definitely shouldn't lose any weight. Between 19.6 and 24.9 is healthy, so you don't officially need to lose weight to be healthy. Over 25 is overweight, while over 30 is considered obese; in both cases you should lose some weight for ideal health.

Medical causes of bloat

While most causes of bloat are harmless and easily fixed, a few may need medical intervention. Having bloat doesn't mean you are suffering from any of these, but you should be aware of them. If you suspect one of the following may be causing your bloat, seek help before trying any of the diets in this book.

Coeliac disease

This affects around 1 in 100 people, and is triggered when the body identifies a protein called gluten (found in grains such as wheat, rye, barley and oats) as a harmful substance and forms antibodies against it. These damage intestinal cells, preventing nutrients being absorbed. This puts sufferers at risk of malnutrition, anaemia or osteoporosis. The main signs of coeliac disease are weight loss, fatigue and diarrhoea – but bloat, stomach cramps and constipation are also linked. If you're suffering seriously from these, it's important to undergo a blood test. If coeliac disease is diagnosed, removing all sources of gluten from your diet will see the intestinal cells recover in a few weeks. You will, however, have to avoid gluten for life.

Irritable bowel syndrome (IBS)

IBS is characterized by erratic bowel habits – constipation one day and sudden rushes of diarrhoea the next. Both of these are usually accompanied by stomach cramps, wind and bloat. Food intolerance can be a common cause of IBS (see page 22), but for some people it is due to an abnormal reaction to the hormone serotonin that triggers gut actions. In this case, a supplement called 5-HTP may help; you need 100–300 mg a day, and if it's going to work it'll show results in two weeks. In others, stress is the primary IBS trigger and hypnotherapy may help. Ask your doctor to recommend a practitioner or visit www.ibs-register.co.uk.

Candida

Every day our body plays host to hundreds of organisms that live in perfect harmony in our system; but, if that harmony is disrupted, problems occur – and candida is one example of this. Higher levels than normal of a yeast called *Candida albicans* develop, leading to symptoms such as mental and physical fatigue, thrush and other fungal infections, and achy joints. The cure for candida is a diet that totally eliminates foods that feed the yeast (including all sugary foods and any that contain moulds and yeasts). On page 59 you'll find a simple home test.

Inflammatory bowel disease (IBD)

This is the overall name for two bowel conditions – Crohn's disease and ulcerative colitis. Bloat is never the main symptom of these, but it can be associated with them. Crohn's disease affects the whole digestive tract and has symptoms including diarrhoea, abdominal pain and sores around the anus. Ulcerative colitis has similar symptoms, but ulcers form along the wall of the colon and rectum. Both conditions tend to develop before sufferers are 40, and the cause is unknown. Control of IBD is via diet, avoiding trigger foods (such as refined sugars, shellfish, wheat and some artificial sweeteners); if you think you're suffering, see your doctor.

Ovarian cancer

In rare cases, bloat can be a symptom of ovarian cancer. If you suffer regular bloat that you can't link to any food or hormonal issue, particularly if you also suffer abdominal cramps that aren't accompanied by diarrhoea, or have incontinence or any abnormal vaginal bleeding, see your doctor as soon as you can. Caught early, ovarian cancer is 95 per cent curable.

Warning

❖ **The information on this page is not intended to replace diagnosis by a doctor.**

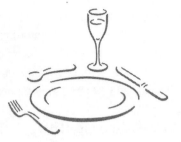

The elimination diet plan

This is the section for you if you ticked mostly Is in the quiz (see pages 12–15) and believe that an intolerance is to blame for your problems. In it you'll find out exactly what an intolerance is and why it causes bloat, try a 14-day elimination diet that aims to reduce your symptoms, and then learn how you can take control of those issues for good – yet still eat the foods that cause you problems.

What is food intolerance?

Food intolerance occurs when a person's body starts to react negatively to certain foods. It differs from an allergy in that food allergies occur when the body interprets something you eat as a hostile invader, and so switches on the immune system to 'attack' the offending item. The result is that within minutes of eating even the tiniest amount of the food to which they are allergic, a food-allergy sufferer experiences symptoms such as wheezing, sneezing, itching, swelling, rash – or, in the worst-case scenario, a form of shock called anaphylaxis, which if not treated immediately can potentially be fatal. Thankfully, only 1–2 per cent of the population suffer a true 'allergy' to what they eat.

Food intolerance is very different. The symptoms of food intolerance are not immediate – they can manifest up to 72 hours after eating a food, making them rather hard to pinpoint. Symptoms also tend not to occur from very small quantities of foods – in fact, one of the reasons why many of the people who suffer from intolerances don't realize they have them is that they only get symptoms when they consume extremely high levels of their trigger food or eat it for several days running; this causes them to attribute their occasional stomach upset or excessive bloat to other factors such as food poisoning or overindulgence. Finally, food intolerance differs from allergy in the sheer number of symptoms it causes. Allergy symptoms tend to focus around the area in which the body is exposed to the allergen – for example, hayfever is caused when pollen is inhaled or gets into your eyes from the air, making your nose and eyes itch rather than your skin –and they tend to be obvious and severe. Intolerance symptoms, however, can manifest in over 20 different ways, affect every area of the body, and range from intense to so mild that you don't realize you're suffering them until you start to look more closely at your overall health.

Exactly what causes food intolerance isn't known. There are, however, three main potential triggers, as described below, and you could be experiencing one or more of them.

Leaky gut

When we digest food, we break it down into small, simple molecules that are absorbed into the bloodstream through the lining of the gut. In some people this lining becomes damaged – this can happen after a cause of food poisoning, because you're lacking certain nutrients in your diet or even during periods of stress. When damage occurs, the food molecules entering the bloodstream are larger than they should be. The body then sees them as invaders and attacks them as it would an allergen. The more often the 'invader' enters the system, the worse the reactions become.

Enzyme problems

Each of the foods we eat needs enzymes to digest it. In the case of intolerance, it is proposed that something interferes with the production of these enzymes; this means that trigger foods can't be broken down and hang around the system for longer than normal, causing bloat and other health problems as they ferment. The most obvious manifestation of this is lactose intolerance. Lactose is a sugar found in milk and other dairy foods, and to digest it we need to produce an enzyme called lactase; many of us just don't produce enough to do the job, however. In some cases this is genetic – 90 per cent of the Asian population produce low levels of lactase, for example – but enzyme production can also be affected by gastrointestinal upsets or stress, or appear with no obvious cause at all. Lactose is one reason why dairy products constitute one of the main groups of foods to which people are intolerant.

While the symptoms of lactose intolerance tend to be linked to clear digestive symptoms such as bloating, pain and stomach upsets that occur within 30–120 minutes of eating lactose-containing foods, you can also be intolerant to another part of dairy – milk proteins, particularly one called casein. If breakdown of this or the other milk proteins is impaired, they pass into the intestine in a partially digested state and irritate the gut lining, causing digestive symptoms including bloat.

Threshold theory

It has been argued that all of us have the ability to develop intolerance to a particular food at a certain level of exposure – our threshold. The threshold varies from individual to individual and no one's exactly sure what controls it. Threshold theory is believed to be one of the reasons why so many people find they have intolerances to wheat. The average person in the UK consumes 50 kg (110 lb) of bread and 3 kg (6 lb) of pasta alone each year; but wheat is also included as a flavour stabilizer in hundreds of other foods – yogurts, soups, soy sauce, crisps and even chocolate can all contain traces of wheat – meaning it has the potential to be in every single mouthful of food we consume. Wheat today also bears little resemblance to that which our bodies have adapted to eating over the last 2,000 years. Modern wheat contains higher levels of substances called lecithins, which are linked to allergies, and higher levels of proteins called 33mers, which are known to be linked to a condition called coeliac disease (see page 18). When people intolerant to today's wheat eat ancient forms that haven't been altered, however, they have no reactions whatsoever.

So now you know the etiology of intolerances, you're probably still asking one final question. Why are they linked to bloating? If you don't have the enzymes to digest a food, it will hang around in the digestive system triggering fermentation and the associated gas. On top of this, a body sees a substance to which it's intolerant as something toxic that could potentially cause it harm; as a result, it tries to dilute it by collecting fluid around it. In fact, the water weight that can accompany a food intolerance can cause people to carry 3–6 kg (6–12 lb) in excess water – weight that disappears when you stop eating the food that causes you problems. This brings us to the diet plan that aims to do just that.

Symptoms of intolerance

✥ Here is a list of the most common symptoms that can be linked to an intolerance to particular foods. You might suffer just one or two, or you might suffer all of them to some degree, but if you stop eating your trigger foods your symptoms will disappear.

- asthma
- blocked nose
- cough
- depression
- dermatitis
- diarrhoea
- eczema
- excess weight
- fatigue
- food cravings
- headaches and migraines
- hives
- joint aches
- mood swings
- runny nose
- sneezing
- stomach cramps
- wheezing
- wind

Day 1

The key to fighting a food intolerance is to remove the potential trigger foods from your diet. In severe cases, this can see people living on a diet so restricted that all they consume is lamb and pears for five days. You're not going to do that; instead, you'll focus merely on eliminating the two foods linked to intolerance in most people – wheat and dairy.

Breakfast

40 g (1½ oz) porridge oats made with **water** or **dairy-free milk**, topped with **3 chopped dried apricots. 200 ml (7 fl oz) calcium-fortified orange juice**.

Lunch

A small can of **sardines** (about 125 g/4 oz) **in tomato sauce** or **1 tablespoon tahini**, served with **4 rye-based crackers** and a **salad** of **baby spinach, sweetcorn** and **cherry tomatoes.**

Afternoon snack

2 handfuls of **unsalted almonds, cashews** or **walnuts**, and any **piece of fruit**.

Dinner

Chickpea and Chorizo Stew (see recipe on page 28), or **quick chilli** made from **125 g (4 oz) lean beef** or **Quorn mince**, simmered with **200 g (7 oz) canned tomatoes** with **chilli.** Serve inside **2 hard corn taco shells** with ¼ **large avocado** and **unlimited chopped onion** and **tomato**.

Do you have a gluten intolerance?

✲ Coeliac disease (see page 18) is not actually a wheat allergy, but an intolerance to a specific protein called gluten found within wheat and other grain-based foods, including barley, rye and oats. Someone with coeliac disease must avoid any products containing gluten for life – unfortunately, this means that this particular diet, which only avoids wheat, is not suitable for coeliacs.

Chickpea and chorizo stew

1 teaspoon olive oil
6 thin slices chorizo, chopped
1 clove garlic, crushed
1 small onion, chopped
200 g (7 oz) bag baby spinach leaves
200 g (7 oz) can chopped tomatoes
200 g (7 oz) chickpeas (about ½ can), drained and rinsed
1 tablespoon fresh coriander, chopped

Serves 1
Preparation time – 10 minutes
Cooking time – 25 minutes

Vegetarian option
❖ Replace the chorizo with a pinch of chilli flakes or paprika.

1 Heat the oil in a medium pan, add the chorizo, garlic and onion and fry for 1–2 minutes, until the chorizo begins to brown and the onions begin to soften.

2 Add the spinach and cook for 2 minutes until wilted and most of the moisture has evaporated.

3 Add the tomatoes and chickpeas and simmer for 20 minutes.

4 Season to taste, then stir through the coriander and serve with brown rice.

Day 2

While the diet here is healthy, it can be hard to get all the nutrients you need when you are cutting out entire food groups, so from today you should also supplement your diet with a multivitamin containing at least the recommended daily amount (RDA) of calcium (700 mg). Also think about taking a supplement of butyric acid, an essential fatty acid that helps repair the gut lining. The recommended dose is about 1,200 mg a day.

Breakfast

Mix 2 tablespoons oats, 1 tablespoon pumpkin seeds, 1 tablespoon almonds and 2–3 dried apricots. Top with 125 g (4 oz) soy yogurt.

Lunch

2 slices dark rye bread spread with ¼ avocado, mashed. Add 50 g (2 oz) fresh prawns, or 1 boiled egg, and sliced red pepper. Serve with 150 g (5 oz) mixed beans, topped with balsamic vinegar.

Afternoon snack

Honey and sesame balls, made by mixing 1 tablespoon sesame seeds with 1 teaspoon honey, dividing into 3–4 balls, and refrigerating for 5 minutes.

Dinner

125 g (4 oz) grilled lamb chop, or 2 Quorn lamb-style grills, served with 200 g (7 oz) mashed sweet potato and a mix of spinach, broccoli and kale served steamed, or sautéed in garlic.

Rye – a great wheat-free alternative

✼ It might surprise you to see a sandwich as lunch today, but dark rye bread, or pumpernickel, is generally made without wheat. Do read labels carefully, though, as some companies make a lighter form of rye bread that is mixed with wheat flour. Rye crackers are also usually free of wheat, but again always read labels carefully.

Day 3

When you're shopping for this diet, you'll notice that you rarely eat the same food more than two days running. The reason for this is that when people give up wheat or dairy they often replace them with another food that they then start to overconsume – this can then lead to the formation of secondary intolerances as you reach your threshold for these too. By varying your diet you avoid this.

Breakfast

1 boiled or poached egg, served with 2 slices dark rye bread spread with a little low-sugar jam, peanut butter or yeast extract. 200 ml (7 fl oz) non-dairy milk.

Lunch

6 pieces ready-prepared sushi and a bowl of miso soup.

Afternoon snack

1 apple or pear, halved or sliced and dipped into 2 teaspoons peanut butter.

Dinner

125 g (4 oz) chicken breast, roast or grilled, or 1 red pepper, halved and stuffed with 125 g (4 oz) butter beans and 2 teaspoons pesto. Accompany with 50 g (2 oz) (dry weight) puy or green lentils (cooked as directed on the packet) and unlimited mushrooms fried in an olive-oil spray with a little fresh garlic.

Quick guide to dairy alternatives

✲ **Used instead of cows' milk on the plan, these can include the following:**

RICE MILK is thin and fairly sweet, and is best used cold as it goes lumpy in tea and coffee.

SOY MILK can contain more protein than cows' milk; it comes in the form of milk, cheese, yogurt and more.

OAT MILK has a neutral taste, so has many uses; it comes in the form of milk, cream and even ice cream.

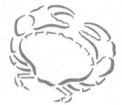

Day 4

Digestive symptoms are some of the first to improve when you remove a food to which you're intolerant from your diet. Even though you've only been on the plan a few days, you may already notice that your clothes are feeling looser around the middle, you're getting less rumbling and grumbling, or aches and pains, in your stomach, and your toilet habits have normalized.

Breakfast

Smoothie made by blending a banana, 2–3 handfuls of blueberries and 200 g (7 oz) canned peaches in natural juice. Serve with 25 g (1 oz) cornflakes or rice cereal with a splash of non-dairy milk.

Lunch

200 g (7 oz) baked potato, topped with 125 g (4 oz) tuna, canned in brine, or 1 hard-boiled egg, both mashed and mixed with a little low-fat mayonnaise. Accompany with sliced tomato and cucumber.

Afternoon snack

75 g (3 oz) tofu mashed with a few drops of vanilla essence. Add 1 teaspoon sultanas.

Dinner

Crab Pad Thai (see recipe on page 36), or make a simple stir-fry with 125 g (4 oz) prawns or tofu and unlimited vegetables (try bean sprouts, bok choy and baby corn) with 50 g (2 oz) rice noodles.

Combining this diet with a family

✷ It's not advisable for anyone who doesn't believe they have an intolerance to follow an exclusion diet; so, if you're cooking for a family, base your meals around the main dishes in this plan but add dairy and wheat products to their meals or snacks, perhaps by accompanying meals with a glass of milk, or putting bread on the table. This is particularly vital for children who need calcium for growth.

Crab pad thai

1 teaspoon groundnut oil
1 clove garlic, finely chopped
2 spring onions, shredded
½ red chilli, finely sliced
a good handful of bean sprouts
1 tablespoon fish sauce
a squeeze of fresh lime juice
50 g (2 oz) medium rice noodles, soaked according to pack instructions
50 g (2 oz) white crab meat
15 g (½ oz) roasted peanuts, chopped
1 tablespoon fresh coriander, chopped

Serves 1
Preparation time – 10 minutes
Cooking time – 5 minutes

Vegetarian option

✲ Replace the crab with 50 g (2 oz) sliced tofu or 50 g (2 oz) extra beansprouts and onions. Replace the fish sauce with strong, wheat-free vegetable stock.

1 Heat the oil in a large frying pan or wok. Add the garlic, spring onions and chilli and fry for 1 minute.

2 Add the bean sprouts and cook for a further minute.

3 Toss in the fish sauce, lime juice, noodles and crab meat, and heat through for a couple of minutes.

4 Serve scattered with the peanuts and coriander.

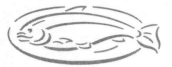

Day 5

If you're finding yourself strongly craving wheat and dairy by now, withdrawal symptoms could be to blame. Both food types contain compounds similar to morphine, called opioids. During intolerance, larger particles of these than normal enter the bloodstream and affect the nervous system, creating feelings almost like a 'high' in your body and withdrawal cravings when these wear off. The cravings will pass.

Breakfast
2 slices rye bread, topped with 50 g (2 oz) soy cheese and 1 sliced tomato, grilled. 200 ml (7 fl oz) calcium-fortified orange juice.

Lunch
Mix 2 chopped hard-boiled eggs or 125 g (4 oz) canned salmon with chopped red pepper and 2 teaspoons low-fat mayonnaise, then spoon the mixture into 2 large lettuce leaves and wrap to eat. Serve with a handful of unsalted nuts.

Afternoon snack
125 g (4 oz) pot soy yogurt and a sliced banana.

Dinner
125 g (4 oz) grilled fresh trout or tuna, or a large flat mushroom stuffed with 125 g (4 oz) tofu mixed with sweet chilli sauce. Serve with unlimited asparagus and potato salad made from 150 g (5 oz) sliced new potatoes and a little red onion mixed with 3 teaspoons low-fat mayonnaise.

Beware sauces and spreads
✣ If you automatically reached for mustard at dinner tonight, beware – some mustards contain tiny traces of wheat or dairy. Other condiments that might also contain them include soy sauce, gravy, Worcestershire sauce, salad cream, ranch and Caesar dressings, stock cubes, tzatsiki, sour cream and hummus. Most other sauces and condiments are fine, but do read labels to confirm.

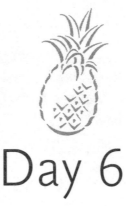

Day 6

Monday is the most popular day to start any diet plan. If you did that, this will be your first weekend day on the plan and perhaps you want to eat out. This can be tricky on any exclusion diet, as you can never really know exactly what a chef puts into his or her dishes, but there are some meals on most restaurant menus that are less likely to contain wheat or dairy products than others (see the list on the opposite page).

Breakfast
Scramble 1 egg, add 50 g (2 oz) smoked salmon or 2 vegetarian bacon rashers, 1 tomato and some chopped spring onion, and mix well.

Lunch
Pizza bites made from 2 rice cakes spread with a little tomato paste. Top with 40 g (1½ oz) grated soy cheese, and 4–5 anchovies or mushrooms, then grill. Serve with a salad of baby spinach, artichoke hearts and cherry tomatoes.

Afternoon snack
Fruit salad made from any 3 chopped fruits, topped with 50 ml (2 fl oz) non-dairy milk or cream.

Dinner
Kebabs made from 75 g (3 oz) cubed pork or 8–10 large olives, alternated with unlimited red pepper, onion and pineapple chunks, all grilled. Serve with 50 g (2 oz) brown rice and broccoli.

Avoiding wheat and dairy in a restaurant
✛ **Choose one of the following:**
- any grilled meat or fish with vegetables and rice, baked potato or chips (French fries)
- stir-fried meat or seafood with vegetables and rice (avoiding soy sauce)
- chicken tikka or tandoori chicken with rice
- tomato-based curry sauces such as rogan josh or jalfrezi with rice
- sushi and sashimi (avoiding the soy sauce)
- any salad without a creamy dressing or croutons

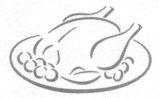

Day 7

By now you may have noticed a slightly unwanted side-effect – an increase in trips to the toilet. This is a sign that your body is eliminating the fluid it has been holding onto. If this is happening, don't cut back on your water consumption – a dehydrated body also hangs onto fluid. Ideally, you should be aiming for at least eight 250 ml (8 fl oz) glasses of water or other fluid a day.

Breakfast

Wheat-free Pancakes (see recipe on page 44), or 2 slices rye toast, topped with 1 teaspoon honey. Serve either of these with a small punnet of blueberries.

Lunch

125 g (4 oz) roast chicken or 2 large slices roast marrow stuffed with a mix of 125 g (4 oz) tofu and 3 chopped walnuts. Serve with 4 roast potatoes (don't use flour to cook these) and unlimited savoy cabbage, carrots and sweetcorn.

Afternoon snack

125 g (4 oz) stewed rhubarb, served with a dash of soy yogurt or oat cream.

Dinner

Niçoise-style salad made from unlimited tomatoes, onions, olives and green beans, and 1 boiled egg. Top this with 5–6 anchovies or a handful of almonds.

Boosting your calcium levels

✳ The biggest problem with giving up dairy foods is that they are normally our prime source of calcium, but plenty of other foods also contain high levels. On this diet we focus heavily on these. They include breakfast cereals, dark green leafy vegetables such as kale or bok choy, fish with soft edible bones such as sardines, salmon, anchovies and whitebait, beans and pulses, sesame seeds and rhubarb.

Wheat-free pancakes

50 g (2 oz) rice flour
1 egg, beaten
100 ml (3½ fl oz) soy milk
a little oil for frying

Serves 1
Preparation time – 5 minutes
Cooking time – 5 minutes

1 In a large bowl, mix together the flour and egg, then gradually add the milk until you have a smooth batter.

2 Heat a little oil in a nonstick pan and add a ladle of the pancake mix. Cook for about a minute, then turn and cook on the other side.

3 Continue with the remaining pancake mix.

4 Serve 2 pancakes as a portion with a filling or topping of your choice, and freeze the remaining pancakes (wrapped in greaseproof paper).

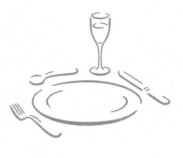

Day 8

If you don't want to lose weight, you're probably wondering if you can drink alcohol on this plan. Wine and cider are fine, but beware – beer contains wheat, as do some gins, whiskies and vodkas. Also, don't forget to stick to safe drinking levels – and ideally have 2–3 alcohol-free days every week. If you're trying to lose weight, however, alcohol is best avoided as it is calorific.

Breakfast

Quinoa porridge, made by adding 50 g (2 oz) quinoa flakes to 2 cups boiling water and simmering for 5 minutes. Add a dash of cinnamon and a sliced banana.

Lunch

2 slices dark rye bread, topped with 2 tablespoons hummus and sliced red and yellow peppers. Serve with a salad of spinach, alfalfa sprouts and celery.

Afternoon snack

25 g (1 oz) plain, salted or toffee popcorn.

Dinner

125 g (4 oz) white fish (try monkfish or sole), or 1 sliced courgette and 125 g (4 oz) butter beans, with 200 g (7 oz) sliced new potatoes (parboil them first), and sliced red and green peppers and onion and a little olive oil, sea salt and rosemary, baked at 220 °C (425 °F), Gas Mark 7, for 15 minutes. Serve with broccoli.

The good grain guide

✳ Until now, you have replaced wheat with common foods such as oats, rice or potatoes, but if you're going to embrace a wheat-free lifestyle and not get bored, or set off a secondary intolerance, you will need to experiment with more unusual grains such as quinoa, pearl barley and buckwheat. The easiest way to prepare these is to boil them as you would rice; whole quinoa takes 15 minutes, buckwheat 30 minutes and pearl barley around an hour.

Day 9

While the digestive symptoms associated with intolerance are the first to improve, by now you should be noticing other positive benefits too. These might be more energy, lack of mid-afternoon sugar cravings, fewer headaches, less congestion or sneezing, and potentially even less achy joints. If you've noticed a decline in any of these things, they were almost certainly caused by either wheat or dairy.

Breakfast

½ **small melon**, topped with **3 handfuls** of **berries**, and **4 oatcakes**, topped with **honey**.

Lunch

200 g (7 oz) baked potato, topped with **3 tablespoons no-added-sugar baked beans** and **2 tablespoons coleslaw** (check labels or make your own with **grated carrot**, **cabbage** and **onion** and a **little dressing**).

Afternoon snack

4 squares plain dark chocolate.

Dinner

Spinach and onion frittata – boil **125 g (4 oz) diced potatoes** until soft, then fry in a small pan with ¼ **onion** until that's cooked too. Add **1 beaten egg** and a **handful** of **fresh spinach** and mix well. Now cook on a low heat until it solidifies. Serve with **unlimited green beans**.

The fructose factor

✲ If you're still getting bloat on this diet, and find it worsens today, fructose intolerance could be to blame. A recent trial at Iowa State University found that 37 per cent of people suffering bloat symptoms had this. Start by eliminating high-fructose fruits (melons, mango, papaya) from your diet, but if it's still occurring try swapping all fruit on the plan for vegetables.

Day 10

It takes about ten exposures to a food or drink for
your tastebuds to truly determine whether you
like or dislike a certain food, so by now you
should have made a decision on regular things
such as having tea or coffee with soy or oat milk.
With other new foods, because you've not yet
consumed them ten times, it may take longer
to determine if you like or dislike them –
but keep trying.

Breakfast
Fruit salad made from 1 sliced peach, 1 chopped apple, a handful of strawberries and a splash of fruit juice. Top with 2 handfuls of nuts or seeds.

Lunch
400 ml (14 fl oz) can any clear soup (check carefully for wheat). Serve with 4 corn, rice or rye crackers spread with 2 tablespoons tahini or low-fat hummus, topped with sliced tomato and alfalfa sprouts.

Afternoon snack
150 ml (¼ pint) low-sugar jelly (made as directed on the packet), topped with non-dairy cream.

Dinner
Cherry Tomato Baked Chicken with Pearl Barley (see recipe on page 52), or roast 125 g (4 oz) chicken breast, or 2 large mushrooms, with a mix of root vegetables and serve with 50 g (2 oz) (dry weight) buckwheat, pearl barley or quinoa.

Where wheat hides
✂ Most of the meals in this plan use unprocessed foods because it's clear that they are wheat free. If, however, you don't like cooking and do want to use convenience sauces or ready meals, you will need to read the labels carefully since wheat comes under many different names. Watch for anything beginning with 'wheat', but also check for bran, bulgar, cereal extract, durum, enriched flour, gluten, kamut, semolina or spelt.

Cherry tomato baked chicken with pearl barley

50 g (2 oz) pearl barley, cooked according to packet instructions
1 skinless, chicken breast
1 tablespoon fresh basil, torn
3 cloves garlic, chopped
125 g (4 oz) cherry tomatoes
2 teaspoons olive oil
100 ml (3½ fl oz) boiling chicken stock

Serves 1
Preparation time – 5 minutes
Cooking time – 40 minutes

Vegetarian option
❖ Replace the chicken with a Quorn fillet and replace the chicken stock with wheat-free vegetable stock.

1 Preheat the oven to 180°C (350°F), Gas Mark 4.

2 Place the pearl barley in the bottom of an ovenproof dish. Top with the chicken, basil, garlic and tomatoes, and drizzle over the oil. Pour over the stock.

3 Place in the oven for 35–40 minutes. At the end of this time, most of the stock should have been absorbed and the chicken will be tender.

4 Serve with unlimited peas.

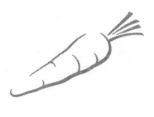

Day 11

If you've decided by now that your problems are definitely intolerance related, you're not alone. The support group Allergy UK believe that 20 per cent of the population suffer intolerance – a figure backed up by a 1994 study published in the prestigious journal *The Lancet*, which found that 19 of 93 patients in a randomly selected group suffered positive reactions to foods commonly linked with intolerance.

Breakfast

125 g (4 oz) prunes (canned in natural juice), topped with 125 g (4 oz) non-dairy yogurt or cream and 1 teaspoon honey. Add 1 tablespoon pumpkin seeds or nuts.

Lunch

Alternative ploughman's lunch – serve 4 oatcakes, each topped with 15 g (½ oz) slices soy cheese. Accompany with celery stalks, some carrot sticks, a few pickled onions and 1 tablespoon sweet pickle.

Afternoon snack

Honey and sesame balls (see page 31) and any piece of fruit.

Dinner

2 fresh sardines or 100 g marinated tofu pieces, grilled. Serve with 50 g (2 oz) quinoa and either 200 g (7 oz) canned ratatouille or your own version made with unlimited aubergines, courgettes and onions simmered in 200 g (7 oz) canned tomatoes.

Proprietary wheat-free foods

✻ Many health stores sell a wide range of wheat-free foods, and they are convenient, but they are also usually highly processed, which makes them high-GI (glycaemic index) foods, meaning that they convert quickly to sugar in your body. A recent trial by Tufts University, USA, linked such foods to true abdominal weight gain, which is associated with a number of health problems and is far harder to lose than bloat.

Day 12

Only three more days to go on the plan. If you're
wavering (remember that you don't get an
intolerance to a food you've never eaten, so if
you're affected by wheat or dairy they were
probably a big part of your life) do a head-to-toe
symptom check of all the things you think have
positively improved since you stopped eating the
two potential trigger foods – and remember they
may come back if you give in.

Breakfast

3 rice cakes or oatcakes, topped with 1 tablespoon peanut butter and a sliced apple. Serve with 200 ml (7 fl oz) non-dairy milk.

Lunch

Mix 200 g (7 oz) canned chickpeas with some diced tomato, finely chopped onion and a little diced cucumber. Add some chopped fresh mint and a squeeze of lemon juice, then top with 125 g (4 oz) chicken or a boiled egg.

Afternoon snack

4 squares plain dark chocolate and a handful of strawberries.

Dinner

125 g (4 oz) any white fish fillet, or ½ sliced aubergine, spread with 1 tablespoon tomato purée and sprinkled with sliced black olives. Bake at 220°C (425°F), Gas Mark 7, for 15–20 minutes, and serve with 200 g (7 oz) mashed sweet potato and some green beans.

Did you know?

✣ The hotter the country, the more likely its inhabitants will suffer from lactose intolerance. That was the finding of a team of experts at Cornell University, USA. They discovered that almost 100 per cent of the population of countries such as Zambia have a problem with lactose, while only 2 per cent of cold countries such as Denmark do.

Day 13

The plan is nearly over and most of your bloat symptoms should have disappeared – if not, and you've already ruled out fructose as a culprit, there may be a more medical reason behind your bloat problems. If you didn't read about these on pages 18–19, turn there now and see if one of these, such as candida, might be affecting you. Candida is an overgrowth of a usually harmless bacterium that leads to bloat and other symptoms after eating foods that feed it.

Breakfast

2 boiled or **poached eggs**, served with a **slice of rye toast** and **2 grilled tomatoes. 200 ml (7 fl oz) calcium-enriched orange juice.**

Lunch

2 corn tortillas filled with **125 g (4 oz) tuna** or **1 boiled egg**, both mashed with a **little low-fat mayonnaise** and some **curry powder.** Top with **1 tablespoon salsa** and serve with **baby spinach salad.**

Afternoon snack

Vanilla tofu (see page 35) with **125 g (4 oz) canned rhubarb in natural juice**, or **light syrup** (drain well).

Dinner

Moroccan Lamb and Cashew Pilaff (see recipe on page 60), or simply serve a **125 g (4 oz) lamb chop**, or **2 Quorn lamb-style grills**, with **50 g (2 oz) (dry weight) basmati rice**, some **broccoli** and **1 tablespoon mango** or **lime pickle.**

Test for candida

✲ First thing in the morning, spit the largest spitball you can into a glass of water and leave it for 30 minutes. If, when you return to the glass, the spitball has turned grey or started to grow 'tendrils', this is a sign that you have an excess of candida in your system (see page 19). Totally eliminating sugar-, yeast- and mould-based foods will eliminate the symptoms, but this is best done with the supervision of a nutritionist.

Moroccan lamb and cashew pilaff

2 teaspoons groundnut oil
½ teaspoon cumin seeds
½ teaspoon ground coriander
125 g (4 oz) lean lamb, cubed
1 small onion, finely sliced
50 g (2 oz) basmati rice
1 cardamom pod
1 cinnamon stick
6 ready-to-eat dried apricots, chopped
25 g (1 oz) cashew nuts, chopped
1 tablespoon fresh coriander, chopped

Serves 1
Preparation time – 5 minutes, plus marinating
Cooking time – 25 minutes

Vegetarian option
✿ Replace the lamb with 200 g (7 oz) butternut squash, cubed.
In step 1, preheat the oven to 200°C (400°F, Gas Mark 6) then
instead of marinating for 30 minutes place the butternut squash
in the oven for 30–40 minutes until tender.

1 Place half of the oil and half of the cumin and ground coriander into a small non-metallic bowl, add the lamb and marinate for 30 minutes.

2 Place the remaining oil in a nonstick pan and fry the onion for 3–4 minutes until beginning to soften.

3 Add the rice, cardamom pod, cinnamon stick and the apricots to the pan, pour over 100 ml (3½ fl oz) water or stock, bring to the boil, cover and simmer gently for 20 minutes until the rice is tender.

4 Meanwhile, cook the lamb under a hot grill until browned and just cooked through.

5 Serve with the rice and scattered with the cashews and coriander.

Day 14

By avoiding wheat and dairy for nearly two weeks now, you will have dramatically detoxed your system of their effects. You may even find that when you get on the scales this morning you've lost a fair amount of weight. The best thing about this diet, however, is finding out what's been behind all those niggling symptoms that have been getting you down – perhaps for years.

Breakfast

Wheat-free Pancakes (see page 44) or 2 slices rye toast, topped with a sliced banana, 2 handfuls of strawberries and a dash of non-dairy cream.

Lunch

Cottage pie made from 125 g (4 oz) lean beef or Quorn mince fried with chopped carrots, onions, 1–2 tablespoons canned tomatoes and some mixed herbs until the mince is browned. Top with 200 g (7 oz) mashed sweet potato, and brown under the grill. Serve with savoy cabbage.

Afternoon snack

1 pear, halved and spread with 1 teaspoon peanut butter.

Dinner

125 g (4 oz) grilled chicken or a mix of shiitake, oyster and button mushrooms fried in a little garlic. Place on a bed of spinach, cherry tomatoes, cucumber and carrot. Add ¼ avocado.

Elisa testing – confirming your results

✵ If you want professional confirmation that you have intolerances, an Elisa test uses a small blood sample to determine whether you possess antibodies to particular foods. If you do, it's a sign that you've had a negative reaction to them in the past, and are either already intolerant or need to watch future intake. A nutritionist can organize this for you, or home-testing kits are available on the internet. These can test for up to 200 different foods.

What to do when the diet is over

After 14 days avoiding wheat or dairy, you've probably realized that while it can be done it doesn't make eating as easy as just grabbing a sandwich at lunch or going out for pizza with friends. Having an intolerance doesn't mean you can't do those things – many people find that as long as they stay under their trigger threshold they can eat their problem food with no symptoms at all. The six steps below can help this happen for you.

1 Work out exactly what your problem food is. Remember that the diet you just followed eliminated both wheat *and* dairy, and you may only need to avoid one of these. The easiest way to tell is the pulse test. When your body encounters a food it's intolerant to, it releases the stress hormone adrenaline in an attempt to speed up your circulation to get the food out of your system; this also speeds up your pulse, so measuring yours can help you spot your trigger food. Sitting quietly, take your pulse, and count the beats for 60 seconds. Now eat a portion of a wheat-containing food, say a bowl of pasta or 2–3 slices of bread. Wait ten minutes, then take your pulse; do it again after 30 minutes, and again after 60. If at any point your pulse rate increases by more than ten beats per minute from that original figure, your body is experiencing stress from the food. If you don't show a reaction to wheat, repeat the test the next day with dairy. If neither shows up, you could be intolerant to something else you also managed to avoid on the diet above – seek professional advice.

2 Try a rotation diet. Most intolerances are only triggered once you overload your system with them. A rotation diet sees you only eating the food to which you react once every four days; in the days in between you choose alternatives. If you don't react, that's an acceptable threshold for you; if you do, then increase the days between your trigger food doses.

3 Look after your gut lining. If your gut lining is healthy, there's less chance of those particles that cause intolerance leaking through. The lining of the gut is one of the fastest-regenerating areas of your body – it replaces itself every four days – and as such you can quickly boost its health by including foods that help heal it in your daily diet. The most important of these are zinc-heavy foods, such as chicken, turkey, seafood and pumpkin seeds, since zinc deficiency is known to slow down cell renewal in the gut.

4 Increase your intake of high vitamin A foods. Foods such as orange and dark green vegetables, liver and eggs are high in vitamin A, which helps repair mucosal linings in the body – and your gut is one of those.

5 Try aloe vera juice. This bitter drink is known to repair damaged epithelial tissue (which includes the lining of the gut). A small glass each morning is normally enough to give effects.

6 Use lactose-friendly products. If you think your problems are definitely lactose related, then either switch to lactose-free dairy products or ask in your local health store for some lactase drops. These are added to dairy products such as milk before you consume them and start to break down the lactose before it enters your system.

The digestion makeover plan

This is the section for you if you ticked mostly Ds in the quiz (see pages 12–15). In it you'll find out why an underperforming digestive system can lead to bloat, find a 14-day plan that aims to 'make over' your system from within, and get some simple steps to follow in the future that will ensure your digestion is always performing perfectly, helping you beat the bloat for good.

Why does a sluggish digestion lead to bloating?

To understand this, it helps to know exactly how the digestion works. The point of digestion is to turn large pieces of food into small molecules from which your body can absorb the nutrients and fuel it needs to do everything it must each day, and it begins as soon as you take your first bite of food. In your mouth, food is exposed to saliva, which contains an enzyme called ptyalin that begins the breakdown of any carbohydrates you've consumed. This and the action of chewing turn the food into a soft paste that you can safely swallow.

After swallowing, food enters the stomach. Here it's exposed to stomach acid and an enzyme called pepsinogen that combine to break down any proteins you've consumed (carbohydrates aren't acted on at all in the stomach). The partly digested blend is further mashed up by contractions of the stomach muscles that you can't feel, but that occur roughly every 20 seconds after eating. After 2–4 hours of this,

'15 per cent of us chew each mouthful twice or less before swallowing, leading to digestive distress. '

a valve at the base your stomach opens, passing the contents into the small intestine where it spends the next 3–10 hours.

Here more enzymes act on fat, protein and carbohydrates, breaking them down into tiny molecules from which nutrients are absorbed and passed into the bloodstream. Whatever's left then passes into the large intestine, where it spends 12–24 hours passing slowly through the 2 m (6 ft) of tubing that makes up this vital body area. During this time, water is extracted and friendly gut bacteria break down the last food molecules until finally anything the body can't use is sent for excretion. If everything is working smoothly, this entire process should take 17–36 hours and cause no adverse side-effects – but that doesn't always happen.

Modern life is the enemy of digestion. At its simplest level, our hectic schedules and constant interruption from mobile phones, for example, mean that most of us rush through meals, and very rarely chew our food well – in fact, one recent study found that 15 per cent of us chew each mouthful twice or less before swallowing. This triggers digestive distress, firstly because it sends food into the stomach in larger lumps than it was designed to handle, and secondly because when it gets there the acid and enzyme mix that's supposed to start acting upon proteins isn't ready (as its release is partly triggered in response to the chewing motion of your mouth). This alone can be enough to trigger bloating, but there are other potential factors involved.

The acidity factor

While the initial release of stomach acid is stimulated by chewing, exactly how much you produce varies from person to person and can be influenced by factors including nutrient deficiency. Stomach acid requires vitamins and minerals for its production, particularly zinc – if you are low in zinc (found in poultry, dairy foods and cereals) you'll also be low in stomach acid. You'll also produce lower levels if your diet is lacking in B vitamins. This is why long-term stress can be linked to low stomach acid production – it wipes out the nutrients you need to make it. Finally, your ability to make stomach acid decreases with age – decline begins in the mid-30s and it is estimated that by the age of 60 half of the population will have suboptimal levels.

Enzyme levels – the second piece of the puzzle

Enzymes are responsible for the breakdown of all of the food we consume, and if your levels are lowered your digestion system cannot function adequately. Most people do have lowered enzyme levels. Again, age is a major factor here – researchers from Michael Reese Hospital in Chicago found that salivary enzymes are more than 30 times stronger in

20-somethings than in pensioners, while German researchers found that stomach-related starch-digesting enzymes were halved between youth and old age. Stress also decreases enzyme production, but potentially the biggest issue is our overprocessed, overcooked diet. Raw foods contain high levels of natural enzymes that supplement the enzymes produced by our body – if we're not eating enough of these we can only rely on our own supplies, which eventually start to run out.

Food-combining to beat the bloat

�֍ **The diet that follows uses the principles of food-combining to help maximize bloat-busting potential. The theory behind this is that eating foods containing high levels of protein and carbohydrates together overloads the digestive system and slows digestion (so they should only ever be combined with vegetables or fats). It's also believed that fruit should only ever be eaten alone. It's a controversial theory, but many people do find that it helps them beat the bloat and so it's definitely worth a try. The first step in any food-combining plan, though, is to know which foods fall into which category – they are not as obvious as you'd think and they vary between food-combining diets. In this plan:**

PROTEIN FOODS include meat, fish, dairy products, eggs, tofu, Quorn
CARBOHYDRATE FOODS include bread, pasta, rice, potatoes, lentils, beans, pulses
FATS include nuts, seeds, butter, mayonnaise, all oils, avocados
VEGETABLES include everything except potatoes
FRUIT includes everything fresh, dried or juiced

Bacteria balance – your last defence against the bloat

By the time food reaches the large intestine most digestion is done, but it doesn't mean that problems can't occur here too. Food moves very slowly through the large intestine (remember that with a sluggish digestion it can be in there up to 24 hours) constantly producing gas as it does this. Gut bacteria, however, stimulate bowel movement, so the more of those you possess the faster things will move and the less gas you'll produce. You may also find that any gas that does develop doesn't cause the sensation of bloat. Recent trials at McMaster University, Canada, found that low levels of gut bacteria were associated with greater feelings of discomfort from intestinal gas.

Creating a healthy gut environment is therefore essential to beat the bloat, and the diet that follows aims to do just that by supplying foods that help increase enzyme levels, boost levels of stomach acid and promote healthy levels of gut bacteria. Follow it for the recommended 14 days and you'll create the optimum environment for digestion – and beating the bloat.

Did you know?

✶ Your gut contains over 500 different types of bacteria, some healthy, some not so healthy. They account for about 1 kg (2 lb) of your bodyweight, but the healthy bacteria can easily be destroyed by things such as a bout of food poisoning, a course of antibiotics or even stress. For optimum good health you need to keep their levels up.

Day 1

This diet begins with something potentially unusual – a glass of water with apple cider vinegar. This is a natural way to boost your stomach acid levels and aid digestion. An alternative is a glass of water containing the juice of half a lemon. Note: if you find you develop indigestion after your vinegar drink, you may have an overproduction of stomach acid and should skip this each day.

Half an hour before breakfast

1–2 teaspoons apple cider vinegar in a glass of warm water.
Repeat this 30 minutes before each of your meals each day.

Breakfast

40 g (1½ oz) porridge oats mixed with water. 1 slice of granary
toast, topped with 1 teaspoon peanut butter.

Lunch

250 g (8 oz) baked potato, topped with 3–4 tablespoons coleslaw
made from grated carrot, cabbage and onion and mixed with a
little low-fat salad dressing. Serve with sliced beetroot.

Afternoon snack

1 slice pineapple or papaya and a banana.

Dinner

Prawn and Spring Vegetable Stir-fry (see recipe on page 74), or
simply top 150 g (5 oz) chicken breast or 2 large mushrooms with
1 tablespoon tomato purée and 50 g (2 oz) grated cheese. Serve
any of the above with unlimited spinach.

Supplementing the diet

❖ The production of stomach acid and enzymes needs a full set of
nutrients, so start by taking a daily multivitamin, but also add a
probiotic supplement. These contain high levels of the good
bacteria you need. For best results, choose ones that say they
contain at least both *lactobacillus* and *bifidis bacterium* but the
more types the better. If you have trouble swallowing tablets, you
could also add a daily bottle of a probiotic yogurt drink.

Prawn and spring vegetable stir-fry

125 g (4 oz) raw king prawns, defrosted if frozen, peeled
2 teaspoons sesame oil
½ teaspoon cumin seeds
1 clove garlic, crushed
1 teaspoon fresh ginger, grated
½ red or green chilli, deseeded and chopped
1 small onion, sliced
6 asparagus spears, halved lengthways (and crossways if they are long)
a handful of mangetout, halved
125 g (4 oz) purple sprouting broccoli
a handful of peas, defrosted if frozen
100 g (3½ oz) shiitake or oyster mushrooms

Serves 1
Preparation time – 10 minutes
Cooking time – 5 minutes

Vegetarian option
✿ Replace the prawns with 125 g (4 oz) tofu.

1 Place the prawns in a small bowl with half the oil, the cumin seeds, garlic, ginger and chilli, stir to combine and set aside for 10 minutes while you prepare the vegetables.

2 Heat the remaining oil in a frying pan or a wok, add the onion, asparagus, mangetout and broccoli and fry for 2 minutes.

3 Add the prawns and their marinade, peas and mushrooms, and continue to fry for 2–3 minutes until the prawns have just turned pink, then serve.

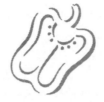

Day 2

Today you'll alter not what you eat, but how you eat it. Chewing well ensures that food enters your stomach in a readily digestible state, and it's recommended that you chew each mouthful 15–20 times before swallowing. As well as beating the bloat, studies at the University of Rhode Island, USA, found that people who do this consume an average of 70 fewer calories at each meal. That leads to a painless weight loss of 3.5 kg (7 lb) a year.

Breakfast
Fruit plate of 2 slices pineapple, ½ papaya and 1–2 kiwifruit. Accompany with 200 ml (7 fl oz) fruit juice.

Lunch
Salad made from unlimited lettuce, green pepper and cucumber, topped with ½ avocado and 4 sun-dried tomatoes. Top with 125 g (4 oz) prawns or 1 boiled egg. Add 1 tablespoon any low-fat salad dressing.

Afternoon snack
125 g (4 oz) low-fat natural yogurt or cottage cheese.

Dinner
50 g (2 oz) (dry weight) couscous mixed with 200 g (7 oz) canned kidney beans, topped with unlimited aubergines, red peppers, onions and courgettes roasted with a little rosemary and olive oil. Add a little sweet chilli or harissa sauce on the side.

Avoiding hunger pangs
❖ Fruit is eaten alone when food-combining, as it is naturally digested quickly. Eat it with other foods and this process slows down and fermentation occurs. However, some people do feel very hungry after meals of just fruit. If you do, add a morning snack about two hours after breakfast. For maximum satiety, make this protein-based such as a low-fat yogurt, 150 g (5 oz) cottage cheese or a boiled egg.

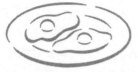

Day 3

So now you're getting a picture of what you should be eating to improve your digestion – but what should you drink? We all need about eight 250 ml (8 fl oz) glasses of liquid a day for optimum health, but when your digestion is weak it's best to drink 30 minutes before or after meals since drinking during eating is believed to dilute the digestive juices. To beat the bloat it will also help if you avoid fizzy drinks.

Breakfast

2 eggs, scrambled, poached or fried in a nonstick pan with a **little olive-oil spray**. Serve with **1 tomato** halved and grilled, and a **handful of mushrooms**.

Lunch

125 g (4 oz) focaccia spread with **2 tablespoons low-fat hummus**, topped with **sliced red** and **yellow pepper**. Serve with a **salad** of **alfalfa sprouts, chopped celery** and **broccoli florets**.

Afternoon snack

½ papaya and **1–2 handfuls of any berries**.

Dinner

125 g (4 oz) fried liver (any kind) or **1 Quorn steak**. Top with **¼ onion**, chopped and fried in a **little olive oil**, served with about **200 g (7 oz) mashed swede** and **unlimited green beans**.

To cook or not to cook?

✲ While it's believed that raw vegetables boost our natural enzyme levels, it's also true that some vegetables are more nutritious if they're eaten cooked: carrots, for example, provide three times more absorbable beta-carotene than raw ones, and cooked tomatoes also release more of the anti-oxidant lycopene. On this plan, therefore, we combine raw and cooked meals equally.

Day 4

One of the first health benefits you're likely to notice when on a food-combining diet is that your energy levels will improve; this is because your body is no longer diverting its energy to your digestive system to tackle foods that 'fight' with each other. You should start seeing the benefits of this now with more energy throughout the day – but particularly during the post-lunch period when you would normally slump.

Breakfast

2 wholewheat cereal 'biscuits', served with 200 ml (7 fl oz) oat or rice milk (see page 33 for more information on these). 1 slice of granary toast with a little low-sugar jam.

Lunch

Salad of 125 g (4 oz) low-fat mozzarella cheese, served with unlimited sliced tomatoes and rocket lettuce and 3 teaspoons fresh pesto sauce.

Afternoon snack

A handful of cashews, peanuts, brazils or walnuts.

Dinner

Butter Bean, Spinach and Blue Cheese Fritters (see recipe on page 82), or a simple stew of 3–4 handfuls of mixed beans simmered on the hob with 200 g (7 oz) canned tomatoes and herbs, served on a 250 g (8 oz) baked potato, with unlimited peas.

Looking after your liver

✿ Your liver is a vital part of the digestive process as it produces bile that helps your body break down fat. When you're trying to improve your digestion, it's therefore important to look after your liver by avoiding alcohol totally – or at least only consuming 1–2 standard drinks a day. A standard drink is 300 ml (½ pint) of beer or lager, 125 ml (4 fl oz) of wine, or 25 ml (1 fl oz) of spirits.

Spinach and blue cheese fritters

1 teaspoon olive oil
½ clove garlic, crushed
pinch of cumin seeds
100 g (3½ oz) fresh spinach
20 g (¾ oz) stilton, crumbled
½ small egg, beaten
½ tablespoon plain flour
pinch of cayenne pepper

Serves 1
Preparation time – 5 minutes
Cooking time – 10 minutes

1 Heat half the oil in a frying pan, add the garlic and cumin seeds and fry for 1 minute.

2 Add the spinach and fry for 2–3 minutes until wilted and all the moisture has been evaporated.

3 Stir through the remaining ingredients until well combined.

4 Brush a nonstick frying pan with a little of the remaining oil. Drop in spoonfuls of the fritter mixture and fry for about 1 minute on each side until golden.

5 Serve with unlimited peas and a crisp salad.

Day 5

You should be enjoying the diet so far, but you may have noticed something about your daily intake – you're eating a lot of pineapple and papaya. That's because these two fruits are a natural source of the enzymes papain and bromelain you need in order to digest proteins and fats. By including them in your diet you are therefore maximizing your digestive power.

Breakfast

Fruit salad made from any **3 fruits** (say **apple, pear** and **strawberries**, or **banana, raspberries** and **orange**), diced or sliced with **1 slice papaya** or **pineapple**. Add **1 tablespoon orange** or **pomegranate juice**.

Lunch

400 g (13 oz) any can- or **carton-based vegetable soup**, served with **125 g (4 oz) crusty granary bread**, topped with **½ avocado**, mashed.

Afternoon snack

125 g (4 oz) low-fat natural yogurt or **cottage cheese** and a **handful of nuts**.

Dinner

125 g (4 oz) salmon, tuna or **trout fillet**, or **1 Quorn steak**, grilled. Serve with **unlimited vegetables** (such as **courgettes, red** and **yellow peppers** and **onions**) roasted with a **little olive oil** and **rosemary** and some steamed **broccoli**.

Enzyme supplements – yes or no?

✲ **As well as all the natural enzyme boosters in this plan, you can further increase their levels by taking supplements. These contain papain, bromelain and another important substance called pancreatin. If you are over 60 and therefore potentially very low in enzymes, you may want to add one of these to your daily diet as well. Take it for a month, by which time your own body normally rectifies levels.**

Day 6

Food-combining is often used as a weight-loss plan, since by eliminating either carbohydrates or protein at each meal you naturally limit your calories. Because of this, you need to eat larger quantities of each food type than normal to ensure you're meeting your daily calorie needs. If you're still hungry after doing this, it's fine to add another snack each day – choose something from the list on the opposite page.

Breakfast

2 slices granary, wholemeal or rye toast, topped with
1–2 tomatoes, sliced then grilled, or 150 g (5 oz) canned tomatoes.

Lunch

Grill 2 large slices of aubergine and spread with a little mustard.
Take 2 slices lean ham and 25 g (1 oz) sliced cheese (if you're
vegetarian, leave out the ham and double the cheese) and
sandwich them with the aubergine slices. Heat for 10 seconds
in the microwave so the cheese melts slightly. Serve with
unlimited coleslaw.

Afternoon snack

1 cereal bar (around 150 calories).

Dinner

75 g (3 oz) (dry weight) pasta spirals tossed with unlimited
wilted spinach, 5 chopped cherry tomatoes and a handful
of pine nuts. Sprinkle with lemon juice.

Extra snack suggestions

- a handful of any nut or seed
- any 2 pieces of fruit
- 125 g (4 oz) pot natural yogurt, fromage frais or cottage cheese
- a handful of vegetables and 1 tablespoon salsa or hummus
- 2 oatcakes, topped with 1 teaspoon peanut butter
- 25 g (1 oz) any cheese with a little celery
- 1 slice pineapple or papaya with a handful of berries

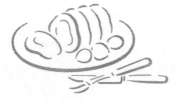

Day 7

Pineapple and papaya aren't the only special foods on this diet – it's also packed with prebiotic foods. These are foods that the healthy bacteria in your diet (such as probiotics) need in order to thrive, and they include oats, onions, leeks, bananas, spinach and beans. In recent studies from the University of Reading, UK, it was found that you can increase your 'bug' levels by over 133 million in just five days simply by eating prebiotic foods.

Breakfast

Omelette made from 2 eggs filled with 25 g (1 oz) grated low-fat cheese and chopped green pepper, tomato and/or fresh spinach.

Lunch

125 g (4 oz) roast pork, or an onion cored and filled with 125 g (4 oz) stuffing mix then roasted until soft. Serve either of these with pea mash (made by mashing boiled frozen peas and a little mint jelly), unlimited carrots and 1 tablespoon gravy.

Afternoon snack

A handful of crudités (cucumber, red pepper, celery) with a little salsa.

Dinner

Indian Lentil and Vegetable Stew (see recipe on page 90), or mix 2 handfuls each of spinach, butter beans and mushrooms with 200 g (7 oz) rogan josh sauce. Serve either of these with 50 g (2 oz) basmati rice.

Enjoy your food

✴ I hope that you're enjoying all of the foods on this diet, but if there is an ingredient that you particularly don't like then do swap it for something else – you could improve your digestion by doing so. Studies from Sweden found that eating a food you enjoy increases the secretion of digestive enzymes and the amount of nutrients you absorb from whatever you consume.

Indian lentil and vegetable stew

1 teaspoon oil
1 clove garlic, chopped
1 teaspoon fresh ginger, grated
½ teaspoon ground cumin
½ teaspoon ground coriander
½ teaspoon turmeric
1 potato, chopped
1 carrot, chopped
100 g (3½ oz) red lentils, rinsed
75 g (3 oz) green beans
2 tomatoes, chopped
300 ml (½ pint) vegetable stock
½ teaspoon garam masala
a handful of fresh coriander, chopped

Serves 1
Preparation time – 5 minutes
Cooking time – 25 minutes

1 Heat the oil in a medium pan, add the garlic and ginger and fry for 1 minute.

2 Add the cumin, coriander, turmeric, potato and carrot and fry for 2–3 minutes.

3 Add all the remaining ingredients except the garam masala and fresh coriander, bring to the boil, cover and simmer for 20 minutes until the vegetables and lentils are tender, adding a little extra stock if the stew becomes a little dry.

4 Stir through the garam masala and coriander, and serve.

Day 8

By now, most people will have noticed a dramatic, positive difference in the amount of bloat they're experiencing – some of you, however, may have noticed an increase. This is because this diet contains healthy levels of fibre and, if you're not used to consuming this, it can take a week or so for your body to adapt. While it does, a cup of peppermint tea will help debloat you quickly and easily.

Breakfast

Blend together a banana, 2 handfuls of raspberries and 2 handfuls of blueberries with a little water or apple juice. Either drink as a smoothie, accompanied by 1 sliced pear and 2 pineapple slices, or pour over the other fruit and eat as a fruit salad.

Lunch

½ avocado, topped with 150 g (5 oz) canned crab meat or tofu, or 6 chopped crabsticks mixed with a little Thousand Island dressing. Serve with a salad of alfalfa sprouts, rocket and green pepper.

Afternoon snack

50 g (2 oz) low-fat feta cheese with 1–2 celery sticks.

Dinner

75 g (3 oz) (dry weight) pasta spirals, topped with 1 tablespoon pesto. Add 5–6 sun-dried tomatoes and 5–6 black olives.

Foods that harm and heal

❊ The foods that help boost good gut bacteria can also create gas in some people, but changing the way you prepare them can help reduce the effects. Beans respond well to being rinsed before cooking, the bloat potential of onions can be lessened by cooking them until soft before adding them to dishes, and the effects of artichokes, leeks and garlic can be reduced by cooking them with spices such as turmeric, ginger or cumin.

Day 9

This plan is based around light lunches, as these are normally easier for people who are working; if, however, you find you respond better to a larger lunch and lighter dinner, there's no problem with swapping these meals around. In fact, according to the theory of Ayurveda (an ancient system of health care native to the Indian subcontinent), we should also be eating our main meal at lunchtime as our digestion is most primed for action at that time.

Breakfast

2 eggs, poached, scrambled or boiled, served with a **handful** of **grilled mushrooms** or some **wilted spinach**.

Lunch

½ **ciabatta loaf** spread with a **little mayonnaise**, topped with **grilled sliced vegetables** (such as **red peppers**, **aubergines** and **courgettes**). Serve with a **salad** of **grated carrot** and **sliced cucumber**.

Afternoon snack

½ **papaya** or **125 g (4 oz) pineapple chunks in natural juice**, served with **2 handfuls** of **any berries**.

Dinner

150 g (5 oz) tuna steak or **cod fillet**, or **1 Quorn steak**, grilled or fried with an **oil spray**, topped with a sauce of **3 medium tomatoes** (or **1 tablespoon canned tomatoes**) chopped with a **handful** of **spinach** and **2 teaspoons capers**, and warmed gently in a small saucepan. Serve with **unlimited green beans**.

Are you sitting comfortably?

✲ **While you're aiming to beat the bloat from the inside, if you're sitting slumped in a chair to eat your meals you could be counteracting your hard work. Research from the University of Medicine and Dentistry, New Jersey, USA, found that slumping slows down the amount of time it takes food to progress into the intestine, increasing the risk of bloat. Sit up straight, ideally at a table, to eat, whenever you can.**

Day 10

As well as beating the bloat by means of this diet plan, by now you might also have noticed that you've lost weight – potentially 1.5–2 kg (3–4 lb). This is partly because food-combining naturally reduces the amount of calories you eat at meals, but also because in order to improve digestion you're also avoiding saturated fats, which your body finds hard to handle, and sugar, which upsets levels of good bacteria in the bowel.

Breakfast

2 crumpets or English muffins, toasted, topped with a little honey.

Lunch

Spicy salad made from shredded carrot and cabbage, some sliced green beans and 2 quartered tomatoes all tossed in a sauce of 1 tablespoon fresh lime juice, 1 tablespoon fish sauce and a little crushed garlic and fresh red chilli. Top with a handful of peanuts and 125 g (4 oz) prawns or tofu.

Afternoon snack

1 pot low-fat yogurt.

Dinner

Asparagus and Artichoke Risotto (see recipe on page 98), or 75 g (3 oz) brown rice, topped with roast vegetables and 5 canned artichoke hearts. Serve either of these with a large green salad.

Are your bowel habits normal?

✻ Because you're increasing the amount of fibre in your diet on this plan, you're probably visiting the toilet more often. That's a good thing – the more stools you pass the lower your chance of bloat. If you're wondering what's normal, however, gastric experts say anything from 4 to 14 stools a week. If you're not reaching even the baseline of this amount, try taking 1 teaspoon psyllium husks in a glass of water each morning to get things moving.

Asparagus and artichoke risotto

1 teaspoon olive oil
1 small onion, chopped
125 g (4 oz) asparagus tips, halved
75 g (3 oz) risotto rice
300 ml (½ pint) vegetable stock, boiling
4 artichoke hearts (stored in oil), halved
1 tablespoon fresh parsley, chopped
plenty of freshly ground black pepper

Serves 1
Preparation time – 5 minutes
Cooking time – 20 minutes

1 Heat the oil in a nonstick frying pan. Add the onion and the bottom halves of the asparagus and fry for 1–2 minutes, until the onion begins to soften.

2 Stir through the rice and coat in the oil. Add 1 ladle of stock to the rice and stir continuously until the stock is absorbed. Continue in this way until all the stock is used up and the rice is tender, adding the remaining asparagus with the last ladle of stock.

3 Remove from the heat, stir in the remaining ingredients, season well with plenty of black pepper, and serve.

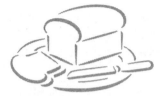

Day 11

By now on this plan the effects of your internal makeover will be showing everywhere – your eyes will be brighter and you'll have fresher breath and clearer skin. You could even find you look younger. When the digestive system is overloaded, people often develop dark circles under the eyes and lines between the eyebrows; as you de-stress your digestive system, these will start to fade.

Breakfast

1 slice papaya, **1 apple** and a **handful of strawberries** all chopped and mixed into a fruit salad with a **splash** of any **fruit juice** or **water**.

Lunch

Sliced pitta bread or **2 slices granary bread**, toasted and served with **2–3 handfuls of baby carrots** and **celery sticks**, plus **125 g (4 oz) low-fat hummus** and **2–3 tablespoons salsa**.

Afternoon snack

2 oatcakes, topped with **1 teaspoon peanut butter**.

Dinner

125 g (4 oz) roast lamb, a **lamb chop** or **6 falafel balls**, served with **unlimited roast vegetables** (such as **courgettes**, **yellow peppers** and **cherry tomatoes**) and a **dab** of **tzatziki** or **hummus**.

Don't overstimulate your system

✲ Because the internal makeover is virtually complete, some people may find they are now suffering indigestion after meals. This is a sign that you're now producing enough of your own stomach acid and that using the apple cider vinegar before meals is overacidifying your system. If that seems to be the case, stop using it.

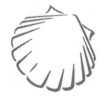

Day 12

So you're nearly at the end of the diet, but you've probably noticed that you're still passing some gas each day. Relax. Even the healthiest digestive system produces about 5 litres (9 pints) of wind each day, much of which is reabsorbed but you will still burp or break wind 20–30 times a day – mostly completely unnoticeably to you (or anyone around you). This wind will also not lead to bloat or cause any discomfort.

Breakfast

2 wholewheat cereal 'biscuits' or 25 g (1 oz) corn or bran flakes (or any other low-sugar cereal of your choice), topped with rice or oat milk.

Lunch

3 stuffed vine leaves (available from delicatessens), served with 150 g (5 oz) ready-made potato salad or tabbouleh and a large green salad.

Afternoon snack

1 slice pineapple/papaya with a handful of nuts and a banana.

Dinner

5–6 scallops, or 150 g (5 oz) any white fish (such as cod, monkfish or sole) or tofu, stir-fried with a little fresh ginger, garlic and chilli. Serve with a selection of steamed vegetables (try bok choy, carrot, broccoli and cauliflower) and a dash of sweet chilli sauce or mustard.

Exercise and digestive health

✴ Although working out won't help your digestion by increasing enzymes or stomach acid, it does stimulate movements of the bowel, helping beat the bloat by ensuring that food moves more rapidly through the intestines. Exercise also helps you eliminate gas; in studies at the Hospital General Vall d'Hebron, Spain, it was found that five minutes of cycling released 27 per cent more gas than simply sitting still did.

Day 13

While your lack of bloat is one sign that your internal makeover is now complete, take a second today to poke out your tongue. According to the theory of Chinese medicine, it's one of the first areas to show signs of a healthy digestion. You're aiming to achieve a tongue that has only a thin white coating and is free of lines down the middle and indents around the sides. If you've got this, you're firing on all cylinders from within; if not, your digestion still needs a little pampering.

Breakfast

½ **papaya,** topped with **2 handfuls** of **raspberries** and a **banana.**

Lunch

1 **veggieburger,** grilled and served in a **small wholemeal roll** spread with a **little mustard.** Top with **lettuce, onion** and **tomato** and serve with **150 g (5 oz) potato wedges.**

Afternoon snack

A handful of **cashews, peanuts, Brazil nuts** or **walnuts.**

Dinner

Oven-baked Ratatouille with Trout (see recipe on page 106), or **125 g (4 oz) gammon steak** or ½ **large aubergine,** both grilled and served with a mix of **boiled leeks** and **broccoli,** topped with **50 g (2 oz) grated cheese,** then grilled. Serve any of the above with **250 g (8 oz) canned tomatoes.**

An acupressure boost

✽ By now you will have dramatically improved the performance of your digestive system but to give it a final boost – or, should you ever need a quick boost after a particularly large meal – you can use acupressure to stimulate digestive movements. The points to press are located on your mid back, around your 11th and 12th vertebrae and about two fingers' width from your spine. Massage these points gently to stimulate things.

Oven-baked ratatouille with trout

2 teaspoons olive oil
1 clove garlic, chopped
1 red pepper, deseeded and sliced
1 courgette, sliced lengthways
1 red onion, chopped
½ small aubergine, cut into small chunks
3 tomatoes, cut into chunks
1 tablespoon fresh herbs
   (such as oregano, rosemary, parsley), chopped
good drizzle of red wine vinegar
1 piece skinless trout fillet weighing about 125 g (4 oz)
few olives
squeeze of lemon juice

Serves 1
Preparation time – 10 minutes
Cooking time – 45 minutes

Vegetarian option
❖ Replace the trout with 200 g (7 oz) canned butter beans or chickpeas, drained and rinsed. Stir them through the ratatouille at step 4

1 Preheat the oven to 200°C (400°F), Gas Mark 6.

2 Heat the oil in an ovenproof tray. Add the garlic, pepper, courgette, onion and aubergine and fry for 5 minutes until beginning to brown.

3 Add the tomatoes, herbs and vinegar to the tray. Place in the oven and cook for 30 minutes, until the vegetables are tender.

4 Place the trout and olives on the ratatouille and squeeze over the lemon juice. Return to the oven and cook for 8–10 minutes until just cooked.

Day 14

So that's it, after today the official plan is over –
and your entire digestion has been improved.
You're now producing higher levels of digestive
enzymes, creating healthy levels of stomach acid,
and probably have the 1 kg (2 lb) of healthy gut
bacteria that every body should possess.
On the next couple of pages you'll find out how
to keep it that way, ensuring that you truly have
beaten the bloat for good.

Breakfast

2 slices back bacon, or **2 frozen hash browns**, grilled well and served with **200 g (7 oz) baked beans** and **1 tomato**, halved and then grilled.

Lunch

150 g (5 oz) poached or **canned salmon**, or **unlimited chopped mushrooms** and a **handful** of **walnuts**, mixed with a **little low-fat mayonnaise**. Serve with a **salad** of **lettuce**, **celery** and **cucumber** and some **asparagus spears**.

Afternoon snack

125 g (4 oz) pot of low-fat yogurt or **cottage cheese**.

Dinner

75 g (3 oz) (dry weight) pasta spirals, topped with **175 g (6 oz) ready-made sun-dried tomato sauce**, a **handful** of **mushrooms** and **6 chopped black olives**. Serve with a **salad** of **spinach** and **artichoke hearts**.

One more reason to quit

✲ If you're a smoker, check the size of your stomach before and after your next cigarette. Nicotine stimulates the nerve endings in the bowel, triggering reactions that can cause bloat or upset stomachs – it has even been suggested that passive smoking can have this effect. If you smoke and regularly suffer bloat, it could be time to consider quitting.

What to do when the diet is over

The great thing about your digestion is that it doesn't take long to make a difference to its health. So long as you don't upset the status quo by getting an upset stomach or taking a course of antibiotics in the next few days, the positive changes you have made will probably stay put for a while. If you want to beat the bloat for good, however, here are some rules you need to remember:

1 Digestion doesn't just occur in your stomach. Don't go back to inhaling your food slumped over your laptop. Even the simple act of taking time to chew each mouthful 15 times will help protect you against bloat in the future.

2 Use 'digestives'. During the diet plan, you had a daily dose of apple cider vinegar to help naturally enhance your levels of stomach acid; as explained, this isn't something everyone should do every day, but there are some more gentle acid boosters that you can include in your daily diet to boost your digestion – these include bitter leaves such as radicchio, chicory and dandelion leaves, and liquids such as Swedish bitters that you can drop in some water to drink before meals. Drinking digestion-friendly herbal teas such as peppermint and camomile can also help move things through the system (remember, though, that it's best not to drink actually with meals).

3 Choose a low-GI diet. One of the reasons the body finds it hard to produce digestive enzymes is that the pancreas (which controls their production) is overworked. The pancreas is where the hormone insulin, which regulates blood sugar levels, is produced in the body. If your diet is too high in foods that cause sudden surges in blood sugar levels (high-GI foods) your pancreas is going to be diverting energy to tackle that rather than your digestion. Switching to a low-GI diet (which includes wholegrain breads and cereals, sweet potatoes, basmati rice and pasta) will help reduce this pressure. See also page 55.

4 Eat some natural yogurt (or take a probiotic daily). Keeping your levels of gut bacteria healthy in this way won't just help your digestion – it also helps protect you against food poisoning, has been linked to lowered levels of obesity, and according to trials at the University of Kheil, Germany, boosts immunity enough to make the average cold last two days fewer than normal.

5 Avoid antibiotics. While they are great at killing harmful bugs, they also wipe out the helpful bacteria in your gut. Many people take antibiotics when they don't need to (colds and flu are one of the biggest reasons people ask their doctors for antibiotics, yet neither of these respond to them) so only use them in emergencies. If you do, always ensure you're taking a probiotic supplement, or including naturally probiotic-filled foods such as natural yogurt with the course.

6 Watch your stress level. The gut is extremely sensitive to emotional issues. Every element of digestion can be negatively affected by stress, from enzyme production through to how fast food is processed through the system and therefore how much bloat is produced. If you do have a high stress load, check out the tips in the section that starts on page 158.

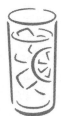

The fluid-fighting plan

This is the section for you if you ticked mostly Fs in the quiz (see pages 12–15). That's a sign that your bloat problems aren't triggered in your digestive system, but in other areas of the body when fluid collects where it shouldn't. For many people, this problem is hormonally linked; for others, it's due to dietary factors and/or a sluggish waste-disposal system. By following this plan, you'll tackle all those problems.

Why you retain fluid and what it does to your system

Water is essential for the health of our body. It makes up around 60 per cent of our bodyweight and we need it to keep our blood flowing, to dilute waste products ready for excretion and to help cool us down by creating sweat. Normally, this fluid is mostly stored inside the body's cells, but about a third is stored within the bloodstream, in the lymph system or in the gaps between the cells, an area called the interstitial space. It's this area that's involved with fluid retention. When fluid retention occurs, the percentage of water contained within the interstitial space increases, which then swells the tissues within it, triggering the puffiness and heavy sensations we know as bloat. As interstitial space occurs in every area of the body, this explains why, when bloat is triggered by fluid retention, it's not just focused around the abdomen but also linked to puffy fingers, swollen ankles and more.

One reason for this incorrect placement of fluid is dehydration (experts at Cornell University, USA, found that 75 per cent of us spend most of our time dehydrated). The body knows that it needs water for survival – in fact, just a 2 per cent decline in your body's water levels can lead to problems such as fatigue, lack of concentration, headaches and so on, while a drop of 15 per cent at some temperatures can be fatal. So, if it doesn't feel enough water is entering the system, your body will start to conserve what it does hold by pushing it into the tissues for storage. Only when you start drinking the amount of liquid that your body needs will it start to release this water.

What we do or don't eat can also contribute to fluid retention: many of us believe that for good health we should be eating high-carb, low-fat diets – but these can actually be the worst thing for fluid retention. Every gram of carbohydrate you eat is stored in your body in three times as much fluid; in fact, many fitness trainers refer to the plump-cheeked look people get when they retain fluid as 'carb face'. Reduce the amount of carbs you consume and you'll also release this fluid.

Low-fat diets are an issue. This is because the membranes of our cells are made up of fatty compounds, but if fat levels in the diet are low these become more permeable, making it more likely that fluid will slip out of the cells and into the surrounding spaces. If you're suffering fluid retention, but also experience dry skin, this is likely to be a problem for you.

> **'Considering the average body needs only 5 g (¼ oz) of salt to provide the sodium it needs a day and the average person consumes 9 g (½ oz), it's no wonder we're puffy.'**

Finally, one of the biggest edible enemies we have when it comes to fluid-related bloat is salt, and the sodium it contains. The fluid that is responsible for bloat is not just water; it's a complex mix of water, minerals, immune cells and more, and your body works extremely hard to ensure that it's kept in perfect balance. If you consume too much sodium, your body tries to dilute this by increasing your level of thirst so you take in more liquid, and by decreasing production of the hormone that stimulates urination. The result of this combination is that you retain fluid. Considering the average body needs only about 5 g (¼ oz) of salt to provide the sodium it needs a day, yet the average person consumes about 9 g (⅓ oz), it's clear to see why so many of us are puffy.

For women, though, there's one final cause of fluid-related bloat that needs to be talked about – hormones. Some women can gain up to 3.5 kg (7 lb) in the days before their period purely because their body is retaining more fluid than normal. Experts even have a name for it now – Type H premenstrual syndrome. It occurs because changes in oestrogen and progesterone levels that occur 4–6 days before your period cause the capillaries of the body to leak plasma into the spaces between the tissues. This alone makes you feel puffy, but the brain also interprets this loss as a threat to your body and slows down the production of diuretic hormones that would normally cause your kidneys to excrete the fluid in your system. While this happens to all women to a certain extent, some become particularly sensitive to the hormonal changes and store higher levels of fluid, triggering premenstrual bloat.

The point of the diet plan that follows is therefore to rebalance the levels of fluid in your body. It's high in foods that promote the excretion of fluid and prevent its retention, but, since hormonal fluctuations are such a common cause of fluid issues in the body, it's also high in specific nutrients that have been shown to reduce the risk of premenstrual issues. Don't panic if you're male – they are nutrients that both genders need for good health, so it won't do you any harm to consume them too. The result is that by the end of the 14 days of the plan you'll find yourself eliminating potentially 6.5 kg (14 lb/1 stone) in excess water weight, beating all your bloat issues, and (for women) tackling some PMS-related issues too.

Did you know?

�֎ You have about 42 litres (74 pints) of fluid in your body each day and it makes up about 60 per cent of your bodyweight. Around 28 litres (50 pints) of this fluid is stored in your cells, and 3.5 litres (6 pints) in the blood or lymph vessels. Around 10.5 litres (18 pints) is the amount normally found in the interstitial space.

Fluid-flushing foods

❃ **LEAN PROTEINS SUCH AS FISH AND CHICKEN** These help your body make a substance called albumin that pulls water from the interstitial space back into the capillaries.

ASPARAGUS A potent natural diuretic, it also contains an ingredient called rutin that strengthens capillaries, helping prevent fluid leaking from these into the tissues.

CITRUS FRUIT The white pith is a great source of ingredients called bioflavonoids that are particularly strong capillary-boosters, again helping prevent leakage.

OILY FISH These are packed with healthy fats that promote the integrity of cell membranes, stopping fluid leaking from these into the capillaries where it can be lost.

BEANS AND PULSES Important sources of the mineral potassium, which opposes sodium in the body – the higher your potassium intake the less fluid you retain.

CRANBERRIES A diuretic food that encourages the loss of fluid from the tissues, they are also packed with flavonols that help prevent leakage from the capillaries.

BRAZIL NUTS Packed with the fluid-fighting mineral magnesium, even just ten Brazil nuts provide you with the 200 mg you need each day.

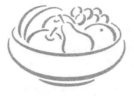

Day 1

This plan starts with some calculations. While the general rule is that each of us needs eight 250 ml (8 fl oz) glasses of fluid (in the form of water, fruit juice or soda, for example) per day to hydrate, this may not be enough for some people. In fact, the specific amount of fluid you need each day is 33 ml for every kilogram of your weight, or your weight in pounds divided by two to get the amount of fluid ounces. See also the advice about exercise on page 122.

Breakfast

125 g (4 oz) pot low-fat yogurt, topped with 2 handfuls of sunflower or pumpkin seeds and 2–3 handfuls of strawberries. 200 ml (7 fl oz) orange or cranberry juice.

Lunch

150 g (5 oz) sliced turkey, or 50 g (2 oz) Brie cheese, served with 1 teaspoon cranberry sauce and salad of unlimited lettuce, chopped apple and pear and a handful of walnuts mixed with 1 teaspoon ranch dressing.

Afternoon snack

Any 2 pieces of fruit and 125 g (4 oz) low-fat natural cottage cheese.

Dinner

Smoked Haddock and Horseradish Fishcakes (see recipe on page 120), or 2 supermarket fishcakes or veggieburgers. Serve either of these with a large stir-fry of bok choy, red peppers, onions and sliced carrots flavoured with fresh ginger.

The tea and coffee myth

❧ It used to be recommended that people fighting fluid retention avoid tea and coffee, as it was believed that the caffeine they contain would flush out fluid, triggering a panic reaction causing your body to hold more. It doesn't. While caffeine is diuretic, it only affects people who are not used to it – and even then the amount of fluid you lose is far less than the amount you take in drinking a cup of tea or coffee anyway.

Smoked haddock and horseradish fishcakes

125 g (4 oz) smoked haddock fillet
300 ml (½ pint) milk
1 bay leaf
2 spring onions, sliced
knob of butter
1 potato, peeled, cooked and mashed
1 tablespoon mayonnaise
1 tablespoon parsley, chopped
1 teaspoon horseradish
1 tablespoon plain flour
a little beaten egg
2 tablespoons granary breadcrumbs
1 teaspoon oil
freshly ground black pepper

Serves 1
Preparation time – 10 minutes, plus chilling
Cooking time – 10 minutes

Vegetarian option

✲ Replace the haddock with 75 g (3 oz) steamed small broccoli florets. Ignore step 1 and stir in the broccoli with the other ingredients at step 2.

1 Place the fish in a small pan, cover it with the milk and add the bay leaf. Place over a gentle heat for about 5 minutes until just cooked. Remove the fish from the milk, allow it to cool a little, then flake.

2 Mix together the spring onions, butter, potato, mayonnaise, parsley and horseradish. Season, then fold through the fish.

3 Spoon into 2–3 patties and dip in a little flour, then egg, then breadcrumbs. Chill for at least 30 minutes until firmed up.

4 Heat the oil in a nonstick frying pan and fry the fishcakes for 3–4 minutes on each side until golden and warmed through.

Day 2

When fluid gets stored in the interstitial space (see page 114), one of the systems used to remove it is the lymph, but sedentary lives mean that many of us have a sluggish lymph system. Exercise, or just simply moving your muscles, will re-energize the lymph, so you should aim to walk for at least 30 minutes a day on this plan. Clenching and unclenching your muscles as you sit will also help move things.

Breakfast

½ grapefruit, topped with 1 teaspoon sugar or sweetener. Serve with 2 eggs, boiled or poached, and unlimited sliced tomatoes, grilled or raw. 200 ml (7 fl oz) cranberry juice.

Lunch

Ham and asparagus roll-ups, made from 3 slices of ham (or cheese) each rolled around 2 spears fresh or canned asparagus. Serve with 400 g (13 oz) any canned soup.

Afternoon snack

10 Brazil nuts and 2 satsumas or other small fruit.

Dinner

150 g (5 oz) tuna steak, grilled or seared, or 1 Quorn steak, topped with salsa made from 1 chopped tomato, ½ chopped orange and a little coriander. Serve with unlimited green beans, sugar snap peas or broccoli.

Body brushing – an extra lymph stimulator

✵ You've probably heard of body brushing, but if you've never done it here are the rules. It should be performed once a day for about five minutes on dry skin. Take a hard-bristled brush, and brush in long, gentle strokes along your arms, legs and torso, always in the direction of either your armpits or your groin (where the lymph nodes are situated).

Day 3

Stand in any health shop and you'll see a number
of diuretic potions claiming to help you fight
fluid retention within just hours – faced with
these, the idea of spending two weeks flushing
fluid may seem a bit pointless. However, most
diuretics release not just fluid from your system,
but vital vitamins and minerals too. Don't give in,
follow the plan and you'll get the same results
with no nutrient loss.

Breakfast
200 ml (7 fl oz) skimmed or soy milk mixed with 2 scoops whey protein powder (any flavour). Serve this with a fruit salad of any 3 pieces of fruit, chopped and mixed with a little orange or cranberry juice.

Lunch
Unlimited sliced red and yellow tomatoes, served with 200 g (7 oz) mozzarella cheese, topped with 1 teaspoon pesto sauce.

Afternoon snack
1 boiled egg, mashed with a little low-fat mayonnaise, served with 2 celery sticks.

Dinner
125 g (4 oz) grilled skin-free chicken breast or tofu, topped with a sauce of 200 g (7 oz) canned tomatoes, ¼ onion and 5 black olives, served with unlimited peas mashed with a little low-fat natural cottage cheese.

The pills you should be taking
✣ Although diuretic supplements are banned on the plan, you should be taking a multivitamin high in calcium and vitamin D. Recent research from the Harvard School of Public Health, USA, found that diets high in these make women 30 per cent less prone to PMS symptoms, including bloat. Taking a fish, or flaxseed oil, supplement to strengthen cell membranes, making them less permeable, will also help.

Day 4

The myth that tea and coffee can dehydrate you has been dispelled on this plan, but alcohol is another matter. Alcohol increases production of a hormone called anti-diuretic hormone (ADH), and when levels of this are high in your system your kidneys are instructed to excrete less fluid and your bloat is likely to get worse. For the next two weeks, try to avoid alcohol totally.

Breakfast

Quinoa porridge (see page 47), topped with **1 chopped orange** and served with a **protein shake**.

Lunch

Caesar salad made from **unlimited lettuce**, topped with **1 tablespoon low-fat Caesar dressing**. Add your choice of **125 g (4 oz) sliced chicken** or **1 boiled egg, 3–4 anchovies** and **25 g (1 oz) grated Parmesan** or other cheese.

Afternoon snack

A handful of dried cranberries and **3 squares plain dark chocolate**.

Dinner

Aubergine and Mixed Bean Chilli (see recipe on page 128), or **2 chicken, pork** or **vegetarian sausages**, grilled, and **200 g (7 oz) mashed butter beans**. Serve either of these with **unlimited steamed broccoli**.

The good news about chocolate

✲ You may find it strange to notice chocolate on this diet plan, but plain dark chocolate that contains at least 70 per cent cocoa solids is a good source of the mineral magnesium. Other good sources, which are also in the diet, are leafy green vegetables, nuts and sesame seeds. Magnesium has been shown to fight fluid retention, as it helps increase levels of potassium in your body. It is also important in helping to combat the sugar cravings that often come with PMS.

Aubergine and mixed bean chilli

1 teaspoon olive or rapeseed oil
1 small onion, finely chopped
1 clove garlic, crushed
1 red pepper, chopped (or half a red and half a green)
½–1 green chilli, finely chopped
½ small aubergine, chopped
½ teaspoon ground cumin
½ teaspoon ground coriander
½ can mixed pulses
200 g (7 oz) can chopped tomatoes
1 tablespoon tomato puree
1 tablespoon fresh coriander, chopped

Serves 1
Preparation time – 10 minutes
Cooking time – 20 minutes

1 Heat the oil in a medium pan. Add the onion, garlic, pepper, chilli and aubergine and fry for 5 minutes until beginning to soften.

2 Add the spices and cook for a further minute.

3 Add the pulses, tomatoes and tomato purée and simmer for 15 minutes.

4 Stir through the coriander and serve.

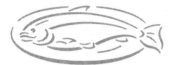

Day 5

You've probably noticed by now that this diet
is high in protein and low in carbohydrates,
and may be wondering if this is safe. It is.
The high-protein diets that cause negative health
headlines are high in saturated fat and low in
fresh fruit and vegetables, which this plan isn't.
Also, because you're drinking plenty of fluid,
you'll be avoiding the dehydration that can make
protein-heavy diets dangerous.

Breakfast

Cheese-topped tomato, made by slicing 1 large beef tomato into 3 slices, and topping each with 1 slice of lean ham, or some sliced boiled egg. Add 25 g (1 oz) grated cheese and grill.

Lunch

150 g (5 oz) canned tuna, or a handful of Brazil nuts, mixed with 200 g (7 oz) canned mixed beans and 1 teaspoon ranch dressing. Serve with sliced red peppers, courgettes and cucumber.

Afternoon snack

125 g (4 oz) pot of low-fat natural yogurt, fromage frais or cottage cheese mixed with 2 handfuls of dried cranberries.

Dinner

150 g (5 oz) any white fish or sliced tofu, sprinkled with Cajun spices and fried. Serve with unlimited roast courgettes, cherry tomatoes and yellow peppers and some steamed asparagus.

The importance of your afternoon snack

✣ If you're trying to lose weight as well as banish bloat on this plan, you may be tempted to skip your afternoon snack to save calories – but don't. When you skip meals, levels of the hormone insulin rise in the system – and insulin can trigger the kidneys to retain sodium and therefore worsen your fluid retention. Eating little and often also helps balance blood sugar levels, which PMS can affect.

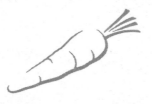

Day 6

Remember that too much salt in your diet increases fluid retention, and it's hiding in some of the unlikeliest places – bread, canned soups, sauces, fizzy waters and even breakfast cereals can all have added sodium – so do read labels carefully to try to keep your levels as low as possible. Also remember not to add salt when cooking vegetables or at the table – this can account for as much as 15 per cent of our intake.

Breakfast

1 vegetarian, low-fat pork or chicken sausage, grilled. Serve with 200 g (7 oz) low-sugar, low-salt baked beans and 200 ml (7 fl oz) unsweetened cranberry juice.

Lunch

400 g (13 oz) chowder-style fish or vegetable soup (from a can or carton), served with a salad of unlimited lettuce, grated carrot and beetroot.

Afternoon snack

5 Brazil nuts and a banana.

Dinner

125 g (4 oz) whitebait, dusted in a mix of flour and a little chilli powder and fried in a little oil spray, or 2 slices of prepared nut roast. Serve with ratatouille made from unlimited diced aubergines, green peppers and onions simmered in chopped canned tomatoes.

You can get PMS on the contraceptive pill

✻ While it does modulate your hormones, if you're on the combined pill that sees you taking a break for seven days each month, you can find that PMS symptoms, including bloat, do hit during that break as you still get mild hormonal fluctuations. Some new contraceptive pills, however, are designed to fight this, so if bloat really bothers you ask your doctor if it's possible for you to change brands.

Day 7

By now, you should have noticed some of the effects of reducing fluid in your system – your stomach, face, legs and hands should all be looking thinner. But you may also notice your cellulite is reducing too – that's because cellulite is a mix of fluid and fat, and by excreting excess water you'll be reducing those dimples as well, particularly if you're using the body-brushing technique (see page 123).

Breakfast

2 eggs, scrambled and mixed with **50 g (2 oz) smoked salmon** or **unlimited grilled mushrooms**.

Lunch

Cauliflower cheese made from ¼ **head** of **cauliflower**, topped with **200 ml (7 fl oz) cheese sauce** (ready-made, or made from **150 ml / ¼ pint skimmed milk, 25 g/1 oz grated cheese** and a **little flour** to thicken), sprinkled with **1 slice of bread** grated into breadcrumbs, then grilled. Serve with **200 g (7 oz) baked beans**.

Afternoon snack

Any **2 pieces** of **fruit** and a **handful** of **dried cranberries**.

Dinner

Crunchy Vegetable and Cranberry Salad with Brazil Nut and Lemon Dressing (see recipe on page 136), or **125 g (4 oz) sliced roast lamb** or **200 g (7 oz) chickpeas**, served on top of **unlimited sliced tomato, cucumber** and **green beans**; also add **1 tablespoon hummus** or **tzatsiki** and a **little harissa sauce**.

Oil on troubled waters

✲ One of the nicest ways to fight fluid retention is to use the power of diuretic aromatherapy oils such as juniper, cypress or fennel (don't use this if you're epileptic). Add 5 drops of your chosen oil to 10 ml of a carrier oil such as almond or grapeseed (you'll find these oils in pharmacies or health stores) and add a splash to your bath each evening.

Crunchy vegetable and cranberry salad with Brazil nut and lemon dressing

1 carrot, peeled
¼ cucumber
a handful of mangetout, halved lengthways
¼ small red cabbage, finely sliced
a handful of watercress
25 g (1 oz) dried cranberries
1 tablespoon fresh mixed herbs (such as coriander, basil and
    chives), chopped

Dressing
2 teaspoons olive oil
25 g (1 oz) Brazil nuts, chopped and toasted
grated rind and juice of ½ lemon
1 teaspoon runny honey

Serves 1
Preparation time – 10 minutes

1 Using a potato peeler, cut the carrot and cucumber into long thin strips, then slice these in half lengthways.

2 Toss the carrot and cucumber strips together with the remaining salad ingredients.

3 Whisk together the dressing ingredients and drizzle over the salad.

Day 8

If you're not getting as much relief from your bloat symptoms as you might like so far, then it could be worth swapping to the vegetarian options on this diet. Research by the Physicians Committee for Responsible Medicine, USA, found that vegetarian diets seem to beat premenstrual-related bloat more effectively than those containing meat.

Breakfast

125 g (4 oz) low-fat natural yogurt or **fromage frais**, topped with a **sliced banana**, a **handful** of **dried cranberries** and **5 Brazil nuts**.

Lunch

150 g (5 oz) canned salmon, or **2 boiled eggs**, mashed with a **little mayonnaise** and served with **unlimited celery** and **carrot sticks** and **2 tablespoons** of **mixed bean salad**.

Afternoon snack

4 squares plain dark chocolate.

Dinner

Prawn and cashew nut stir-fry, made by frying **125 g (4 oz) prawns, tofu** or **Quorn** with **unlimited bok choy, bean sprouts, broccoli** and **baby corn** with a **little garlic, lemon** and **chilli**. Top with a **handful** of **cashew nuts**.

The simple move that flushes fluid

✲ **Anything that stimulates the kidneys will help increase the amount of fluid you lose on this plan, and one simple move that works is the seated spinal twist. Sit on the floor and cross your left leg over your right. Now reach your left arm as far around and behind you as you can and twist your torso so you're looking over your right shoulder. Hold for five deep breaths. Do this once on each side, once a day.**

Day 9

If you haven't been watching your weight yet on this plan, take a few seconds today to calculate your body mass index (see page 17). Because body fat is actually an oestrogen-producing substance (and high oestrogen can trigger excess fluid), the more you have, the higher your bloat potential. If your BMI is over 25, you may want to think about reducing portion sizes.

Breakfast

125 g (4 oz) low-fat natural cottage cheese, served with ½ mango, sliced, a handful of strawberries and a handful of walnuts. 200 ml (7 fl oz) cranberry juice.

Lunch

Greek-style salad made from cucumber, red onion, sliced tomato and 5 olives, topped with 125 g (4 oz) low-fat feta cheese. Add 1 tablespoon low-fat vinaigrette.

Afternoon snack

5 Brazil nuts and a handful of dried cranberries.

Dinner

125 g (4 oz) steak, or 1 Quorn steak, grilled and served with 150 g (5 oz) canned refried beans. Add ½ avocado and 2 tablespoons low-fat coleslaw, or make your own by grating unlimited carrot, white cabbage and red onion and mixing with 1 tablespoon any low-calorie dressing.

Light up your life

✵ Going outside today could help you fight fluid-related bloat. In studies published in the journal *Psychiatry Research*, people exposed to bright light suffered fewer feelings of sadness, irritability, fatigue and bloat than those who were not brightening up their world. It takes about 15 minutes of natural light to get results. In summer, early-morning light is powerful enough; in winter, midday rays are the most helpful.

Day 10

By now, you've probably lost about 75 per cent of the excess fluid you were carrying fairly easily and already feel as if you've beaten most of your bloat. The last few litres are potentially the hardest to lose, so from now on you'll be eating extra high levels of naturally diuretic vegetables: these include artichokes, asparagus, onions, celery and cucumber.

Breakfast

200 ml (7 fl oz) skimmed milk blended with **2 scoops whey protein powder** and **2 handfuls of strawberries**. Serve with a **sliced banana** and a **handful of nuts or seeds**.

Lunch

Antipasto-style plate of **4 stuffed vine leaves, unlimited canned artichoke hearts, 5–6 olives** and **75 g (3 oz) parma ham** or **low-fat feta cheese**.

Afternoon snack

3 celery sticks, served with **2 soft-cheese triangles**.

Dinner

Spring Vegetable Poached Chicken (see recipe on page 144), or **125 g (4 oz) grilled chicken breast**, topped with **2 teaspoons pesto**, or **1 red pepper halved** and stuffed with **2 tablespoons cannellini beans mixed with pesto**. Serve any of these with **unlimited red cabbage** and **asparagus**.

How liquid is your diet?

✲ You take in about 750 ml (1¼ pints) of liquid from the food you eat each day. While the fluid content of juicy foods such as fruit and vegetables is clearly high, it might surprise you to find out how much liquid other foods contain. Boiled potatoes are 80 per cent water, bananas are 75 per cent water, eggs are 74 per cent water, and even dried fruit such as all those cranberries are 20 per cent water.

Spring vegetable poached chicken

1 boneless, skinless chicken breast
1 bay leaf
6 new potatoes, halved
1 carrot, chopped
1 stick celery, chopped
2 shallots, peeled
300 ml (½ pint) chicken stock
100 g (3½ oz) asparagus
100 g (3½ oz) peas
freshly ground black pepper

Serves 1
Preparation time – 10 minutes
Cooking time – 30 minutes

Vegetarian option
✵ Replace the chicken with a Quorn fillet and replace the chicken stock with vegetable stock.

1 Place the chicken, bay leaf, potatoes, carrot, celery and shallots in a medium pan. Pour over the stock, bring to the boil, season, cover and simmer for 25 minutes.

2 Add the remaining ingredients and cook for a further 5 minutes.

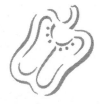

Day 11

Increasing the amount of movement you do each day will help fight fluid retention, but from today you can also help reduce lymph stagnation by being careful about how you sit. Crossing your legs or slumping in your chair both reduce lymph movement, as does wearing tight clothing. Keep things loose and sit upright with both feet on the floor for the rest of the week.

Breakfast

Quinoa porridge (see page 47), topped with **5–6 canned prunes in natural juice** and a **handful** of **dried cranberries.**

Lunch

Salad made from **unlimited ribbons of carrot, celery, cucumber** and **courgette,** topped with **125 g (4 oz) sliced turkey** or **2 handfuls of walnuts.** Add **1 tablespoon** any **low-calorie salad dressing** or **2 tablespoons salsa.**

Afternoon snack

200 ml (7 fl oz) skimmed milk mixed with **2 scoops whey protein powder** and blended with **2–3 handfuls of blueberries** and a **banana.**

Dinner

150 g (5 oz) salmon, or **6 balls falafel,** grilled. Accompany with **1 tablespoon salsa** or **tzatziki** and serve with **unlimited asparagus** and **sliced grilled red pepper.**

Bored with your current exercise regime?

✲ **Try rebounding. Many natural health experts believe that this workout, where you jump up and down on a mini-trampoline, is the ultimate exercise to stimulate lymph movement and therefore flush out fluid. All it takes to get results is five minutes of jumping three times a day. Skipping will have a similar effect, but it's harder on your joints.**

Day 12

You should already be pleased with your results
by this stage of the plan, but for a final 'power-up'
add 2–3 cups of dandelion tea into your routine
for the last three days. A natural diuretic, it's safe
to use because it doesn't trigger any nutrient
loss when you drink it, but it will flush out any
final excesses – you'll find dandelion teabags
in health stores. Brew for 1–2 minutes.

Breakfast
125 g (4 oz) low-fat yogurt or cottage cheese, topped with
5–6 prunes, 1 sliced orange and 6 Brazil nuts.

Lunch
400 g (13 oz) can or carton any bean- or lentil-based soup,
served with a salad of unlimited rocket, celery and cucumber
with 6 sun-dried tomatoes and 5 black olives.

Afternoon snack
A handful of grapes or strawberries and 50 g (2 oz) any cheese.

Dinner
1 low-fat beefburger or veggieburger, grilled well, topped
with sliced onion, tomato and ¼ avocado. Serve with roasted
parsnip – cut ½ large parsnip into wedge shapes, boil for
5 minutes until softened, then roast at 200°C (400°F), Gas Mark 6,
for 25–30 minutes – and 2 tablespoons low-fat coleslaw.

Has your doctor caused your bloat?
✲ Just as the contraceptive pill can be related to fluid retention, so
can a number of other medications, including anti-inflammatory
painkillers, hormone replacement therapy (HRT) and steroids. In
most cases, the problem will be mild – and taking other steps such
as reducing sodium will counteract it; if you're suffering from
extreme fluid issues, however, ask your doctor if there are other
options. Never stop taking any medication without advice.

Day 13

When you first started this diet, you probably found that many of the foods within it tasted bland without salt. After ten days of avoiding something, though, you will stop missing it and that's now what has happened to you. In fact, if you were to add salt to your lunch today (which isn't recommended or you'll regain some of the water weight already lost) you would probably find it totally unpalatable.

Breakfast

200 g (7 oz) kipper, grilled, or **200 g (7 oz) low-sugar, low-salt baked beans,** served with **unlimited grilled tomatoes** or **mushrooms. 200 ml (7 fl oz) cranberry juice.**

Lunch

Asparagus frittata, made by mixing **2 eggs, 4 spears canned asparagus** and **¼ onion** (already softened by gentle frying) in a large frying pan, then slowly grilling until the mixture firms. Serve with a **salad** of **unlimited rocket** and **3–4 sun-dried tomatoes.**

Afternoon snack

4 squares plain dark chocolate and a **banana.**

Dinner

Garlic and Basil Thai Chicken (see recipe on page 152), or any **350-calorie vegetable curry ready meal** (no rice) served with **wilted spinach.**

Increasing your fruit and vegetable intake

✲ On this plan, you're often eating more than the recommended five portions of fruit and vegetables a day. This is partly to ensure you're getting the high levels of flavonols you need to keep your capillaries strong, but also to boost your fibre levels in the absence of carbohydrates. Fibre is also an important weapon in fighting fluid retention, since it absorbs moisture.

Garlic and basil Thai chicken

1 teaspoon oil
1 boneless, skinless chicken breast, sliced
1 clove garlic, crushed
3 spring onions, chopped
½ green chilli, sliced
a handful of fresh basil
grated rind and juice of ½ lime
1 teaspoon fish sauce
100 ml (3½ fl oz) coconut milk

Serves 1
Preparation time – 10 minutes
Cooking time – 8 minutes

Vegetarian option
✤ Replace the chicken with 125 g (4 oz) chopped tofu and
the fish sauce with half a crumbled vegetable stock cube.

1 Heat the oil in a frying pan, add the chicken and garlic and fry for 2–3 minutes until the chicken begins to brown.

2 Add the spring onions, chilli and basil and continue to fry for 2 minutes.

3 Stir in the remaining ingredients and simmer for a further 2 minutes.

4 Serve with steamed rice or noodles and unlimited stir-fried vegetables.

Day 14

So now you've nearly finished the plan, and if you stand on the scales today you'll find you've lost 1.5–3.5 kg (3–7 lb) of water weight (plus potentially 0.5–1 kg/1–2 lb of actual fat caused by reducing your calories). You'll also find that you've dropped up to 5 cm (2 inches) around your waist, plus up to 2.5 cm (1 inch) from each thigh. To ensure that things stay this way, see pages 156–157.

Breakfast

1 egg, poached, scrambled or fried with a little oil spray, served with 2 slices of pork, turkey or vegetarian bacon, well grilled, and 2 handfuls of wilted spinach. 200 ml (7 fl oz) cranberry juice.

Lunch

Salad of unlimited celery, apple and lettuce, topped with 1 tablespoon raisins, a handful of walnuts and 50 g (2 oz) Stilton cheese.

Afternoon snack

1 orange and 5 Brazil nuts.

Dinner

125 g (4 oz) roast pork, or 2 slices of ready-made nut roast, served with 1 tablespoon low-sugar apple sauce, unlimited cabbage, carrots and peas, and 1 tablespoon gravy.

The perfect fluid balance

✲ Assuming all has gone well with your plan, your body should now be losing and gaining fluid in the perfect balance for health. As a general rule, you take in 2.6 litres (4½ pints) of fluid each day through food and drink, and lose the same amount through sweat from your skin (around 600 ml/1 pint), air from your lungs (400 ml/14 fl oz), urine excreted by the kidneys (1.5 litres/2½ pints) and just 100 ml (3½ fl oz) through your bowels.

What to do when the diet is over

You've now eliminated as much excess fluid as possible from your body and should be happily admiring your new svelte shape in the mirror, but how can you help it stay that way? These six steps are what you need to know to make it happen.

1 Keep drinking your personal water prescription (see page 118). Remember, also, that you may need more fluid than even this if the weather is hot or you are exercising intensely. As a general guide, if your urine is darker than a light straw colour then you aren't taking in as much fluid as your body needs, and you should drink some more.

2 When you drink, sip rather than guzzle. A strange cause of dehydration is drinking the liquid you consume too fast. When you do this, it causes a sudden increase in your blood volume, which your body sees as a negative thing, triggering it to release higher than normal levels of diuretic hormones – the result is that you'll spend the next 30 minutes nipping to and from the toilet losing everything you've just put in.

3 Remember that alcohol is a generally a diuretic. If you drink it, you will suffer symptoms of dehydration such as dry mouth, headaches or a hangover, followed by extra puffiness as your body tries to hold on to fluid that it thinks it's at risk of losing. The exception to this rule, though,

> ‘If your urine is darker than a light straw colour you aren't taking in as much fluid as your body needs.’

are beers that contain less than 4 per cent alcohol; with these, the amount of fluid you consume counteracts any effects of the alcohol. If you do want to drink alcohol, sticking to lower-alcohol beers will help fight the fluid-retaining effects the day after. If you drink anything else, alternating a glass of water for every alcoholic drink will also help rebalance fluid in and fluid out.

4 Increase your level of zinc-heavy foods. You should have realized over the last 14 days that you don't need salt to make food taste good, and that focusing on the taste of fresh vegetables or using herbs and spices is better than covering everything with one flavour. If, however, you're not feeling satisfied with the flavours of the food you eat, it might help to increase the levels of zinc-heavy foods (such as shellfish, nuts and seeds) in your diet. Zinc helps boost the activity of tastebuds.

5 Keep an eye on your salt levels. Sometimes, if someone else is cooking, or if you go out for dinner or succumb to a fast-food takeaway you can't control how much salt is in a meal. So, to reduce the risk of bloat the next day, increase your intake of potassium-rich foods, which encourage your body to flush sodium out of the system. Bananas, orange juice and potatoes are all high in potassium.

6 Keep up the high calcium intake and get some sunshine. When the sun's rays hit our skin, they trigger the production of vitamin D, which the body needs to adequately absorb that calcium you're consuming. In fact, if your vitamin D levels are high, you'll absorb nine times more calcium than you will if you're lacking it. You only need 15 minutes of sunshine a day to get results.

The stress-fighting plan

This is the section for you if you ticked mostly Ss in the quiz (see pages 12–15). This means that your bloat problems are likely to be related to your stress load and hectic life. It may seem like an unusual link, but there are many reasons why stress and bloat are connected. In the pages that follow you'll determine exactly what they are and how to deal with them.

How stress can be behind your bloat

Your emotions and your digestion are so strongly linked that the gut area has been named the 'second brain' by researchers. When you are suffering from stress, your digestion can alter in a number of ways that can lead to bloat being triggered. The first is that under stress digestion slows down. This is a throwback to the days when stress meant that something – perhaps a sabre-toothed tiger – was going to attack you and that unless you ran fast in the opposite direction you were in trouble. To do this effectively, you needed a ready supply of blood to your muscles and so blood was moved from other areas, such as the stomach, slowing digestion. Exactly the same thing happens to us nowadays, but potentially for days at a time as we suffer long-term stress, leading to constant digestive deprivation and a sluggish system. When digestion slows down, food ferments and gas occurs, together with the bloat it causes.

Secondly, stress also has a negative impact on digestion because it interferes with the substances you need to carry it out – particularly stomach acid. In trials at the Universiti Kebangsaan, Malaysia, it was found that, during times of stress, levels of gastric acid fell by 40 per cent. This happens because during stress the body shuts down any function not linked to your immediate survival – and, as most of us don't tend to eat while fleeing, the production of stomach acid falls into this category. Stress has also been found to negatively affect the levels of healthy bacteria in the large intestine; these control the movement of food through the gut during the final stages of digestion, and if their numbers are depleted things get sluggish and bloat occurs. During stress, however, chemicals released cause the unhealthy bacteria in your body to turn on the healthy bacteria they normally contentedly co-exist with, leading to destruction and lower levels of the latter in your body.

Hurried lives also mean bloated bellies

Stress can also cause bloat because when we're under pressure we tend to ignore our healthy nutritional needs, reaching instead for sugary and fatty foods. Fat is linked to bloat because the body finds it hard to digest, which slows down the process of food through your system. Sugar is a bloat causer since it feeds unhealthy bacteria that live in the gut, and when these flourish bloat occurs. Finally, during stress we tend to eat faster than normal – the average lunchbreak is now 14 minutes and 27 seconds, and even that is decreased when we're under pressure – and the faster we eat the more air we swallow. That air then triggers bloat. That's assuming we eat at all – 39 per cent of people say they skip meals when they're under pressure; when we skip meals, the body 'panics' and produces higher than normal levels of stress hormones, and this can lead to further problems.

> '**The average lunch break is now 14 minutes and 27 seconds and even that is decreased when we're under pressure.**'

The cortisol connection

One of the main hormones released when the body is under stress is cortisol. One effect its release has in the body is the retention of fluid, so, as well as dealing with gas-related bloat, you'll be experiencing fluid issues. Cortisol also depletes levels of the minerals calcium and magnesium in your system. These are both calming nutrients, and if their levels are low you'll be more likely to feel stress symptoms – creating a vicious circle of anxiety and irritation and all the digestive symptoms that come with them. The point of the diet plan that follows is therefore threefold: it helps you eat in a way that's conducive to lowering levels of stress hormones in the body; it strengthens your body's ability to cope with any pressure it finds itself under; and it also aims to give you tactics that help you fight stress. There's no point in eating a de-stressing diet if you don't also reduce the amount of pressure you're experiencing, so this plan is as much of a mental makeover as a dietary one. You'll find that using the psychological tips and tricks provided within it will boost the effects of the diet and maximize your bloat-beating potential.

Stress and true weight gain

�֎ Stress doesn't just lead to bloating, it can also cause true weight gain around the abdomen. The culprit here is also cortisol. As well as all the other negative effects that cortisol can have on your digestive system, it is an appetite stimulator, and particularly triggers cravings for high-fat, high-sugar foods that your body feels it needs to fuel the fight against whatever is causing the stress. If you're living in a case of permanent stress and cortisol release, you will potentially be eating more calories than you normally would – and those calories will also be more readily stored. Cortisol also seems to have a role in shuttling excess calories into the fat stores of the abdomen.

The ultimate calming foods

❊ BANANAS High in tryptophan, bananas are also packed with vitamin B6, which our body needs in order to manufacture the calming hormone serotonin.

BLUEBERRIES Very high in vitamin C, and German researchers have found that when vitamin C levels in the blood are high we calm down from stress much more rapidly than when they're low.

BROCCOLI High in the mineral chromium. This is good for two reasons: it helps balance blood sugar levels, and increases the amount of tryptophan that reaches the brain.

CHOCOLATE Not only does it traditionally make us feel good, but it also contains an ingredient called anadamide, which has a calming effect on the brain.

NUTS AND SEEDS Some of the best sources of the calming mineral magnesium. Magnesium helps with mental relaxation, but also acts on the muscles helping fight the tension that often comes with stress.

OATS Oats contain ingredients known for their ability to calm the nervous system during periods of stress. In herbal medicine, this ingredient is known as *avena sativa*, the botanical name for oats.

OILY FISH These are packed with high levels of docosahexaenoic acid (DHA) that regulates emotions, meaning you're less likely to stress over little things.

ONIONS These contain high levels of a substance called quercetin that calms the nervous system.

TURKEY A good source of an amino acid called tryptophan, which the body converts into its number one relaxing neurotransmitter, serotonin.

Day 1

This diet is based on the principle of eating little and often, which helps fight stress because it regulates blood sugar levels, improving your moods and your ability to deal with what life throws at you. Too long between meals triggers your body to produce higher levels of cortisol and other stress hormones, increasing agitation. Ideally, you should eat every 3–4 hours during the day; if you have a long gap between breakfast and lunch, choose 1–2 items from the breakfast menu for a mid-morning snack.

Breakfast

40 g (1½ oz) porridge oats made with water. Add **1 teaspoon raisins** and top with a **sliced banana**. **1 orange** and **1 small handful of pumpkin** or **sunflower seeds** or small nuts such as **cashews** or **almonds**.

Lunch

2 slices rye or **granary toast**, topped with **125 g (4 oz) can sardines (in brine or tomato sauce)**, or **½ mashed avocado**, topped with **sliced yellow peppers** and **alfalfa sprouts**, served with a **salad** of **carrot, onion** and **cucumber**.

Afternoon snack

4 squares plain dark chocolate.

Dinner

Warm Salmon, Lentil, Broad Bean and Toasted Seed Salad (see recipe on page 166), or **125 g (4 oz) grilled salmon steak**, or **1 Quorn steak**, served with **150 g (5 oz) boiled new potatoes** and **unlimited steamed broccoli**.

Time to get moving

✲ While exercise plays a role in most of the plans in this book, it's absolutely essential for people who have stress as their primary bloat trigger. Exercise dramatically helps lower stress levels in the body by burning off the high levels of adrenaline in your system that are making you jittery. It also gives you time to yourself. Aim for at least three 30-minute sessions of exercise (and that could be as easy as a brisk walk) a week on this plan.

Warm salmon, lentil, broad bean and toasted seed salad

2 teaspoons olive oil
1 clove garlic, crushed
2 spring onions, sliced
½ can green lentils, drained and rinsed
75 g (3 oz) broad beans, cooked and skinned
8 cherry tomatoes, halved
a handful of watercress, torn
1 tablespoon toasted mixed seeds (such as pumpkin
   and sunflower)
2 teaspoons balsamic vinegar
125 g (4 oz) salmon fillet, skinned

Serves 1
Preparation time – 10 minutes
Cooking time – 5 minutes

Vegetarian option
✣ Replace the salmon with an extra 100g (3½ oz) broad beans
and toss some rocket through the salad before serving.

1 Heat the oil in a nonstick frying pan. Add the garlic and spring onions and fry for a minute.

2 Add the lentils and broad beans and warm through. Remove from the heat and stir through the tomatoes, watercress, seeds and balsamic vinegar.

3 Meanwhile, place the salmon in a nonstick frying pan and cook for 2–3 minutes on each side.

4 Flake the salmon and toss through the salad.

Day 2

On this diet, try to steer clear of excessive amounts of caffeine; studies at Duke University, North Carolina, US have found it increases levels of stress hormones in the body. Two or three cups of coffee or cola a day won't hurt, but if you normally consume more than that cut down by adding a little more decaff to each cup. If you get withdrawal symptoms such as headaches, the homeopathic remedy called 'coffea crudea' can reduce them.

Breakfast

1 crumpet, toasted, topped with **1 teaspoon low-sugar blueberry** (or other) **jam. 200 ml (7 fl oz) freshly squeezed**, or **calcium-enriched, orange juice. 1 apple** or **pear**, sliced and dipped into **2 teaspoons peanut butter**.

Lunch

Unlimited crudités of **celery, carrot** and **broccoli florets** dipped into **150 g (5 oz) low-fat hummus** or **125 g (4 oz) taramasalata**.

Afternoon snack

3 oatcakes or **rye crackers**, topped with a **mashed banana**.

Dinner

125 g (4 oz) lean steak, or **150 g (5 oz) cubed tofu**, sliced and fried with **unlimited onions, red** and **green peppers** and a **little fresh chilli**. Serve in **1 wholemeal tortilla wrap**, accompanied by **50 g (2 oz) (dry weight) basmati rice** and **1 tablespoon salsa**.

Herbal helpers

✲ If you're looking for something to replace your morning coffee habit, energizing herbal teas such as ginger or a shot of dandelion coffee will give you a natural internal boost without increasing your levels of stress hormones. However, the most important herbal tea to introduce to your diet is camomile. Not only is this an important nerve tonic, but it also helps stimulate digestion, fighting bloat at its source. Camomile is a sedative so it is best drunk in the evening.

Day 3

As well as working on a little-and-often approach, this diet is also a low-GI plan (see page 55), using wholegrain cereals, basmati rice and sweet potatoes over say white bread, white rice and normal potatoes to further balance blood sugar levels. If a specific variety of carbohydrate (such as rye bread or bran cereal) is mentioned, it's for GI balancing reasons, so do try to follow these suggestions.

Breakfast
125 g (4 oz) pot low-fat yogurt (any flavour), topped with a handful of walnuts and a handful of blueberries. 1 slice malt loaf with a little low-fat spread.

Lunch
200 g (7 oz) baked potato, topped with 2 tablespoons coleslaw and 150 g (5 oz) baked beans. Add a small salad of lettuce, cucumber and tomato.

Afternoon snack
2 squares plain dark chocolate and a banana.

Dinner
125 g (4 oz) turkey breast, or a large Portabella mushroom, grilled and served with unlimited roast vegetables (try aubergines, green peppers and mushrooms) with roast parsnip – cut ½ large parsnip into wedge shapes, boil for 5 minutes until softened, then roast at 200°C (400°F), Gas Mark 6, for 25–30 minutes.

How carbohydrates fight stress
✻ They provide energy and stress-fighting B vitamins, as well as helping your body produce the calming neurotransmitter serotonin. In fact, wholegrain carbs will give your body a shot of serotonin in as little as 30–45 minutes – eating protein with carbs slows this reaction, which is why many of the meals on this plan are high in carbs and vegetables but low in protein.

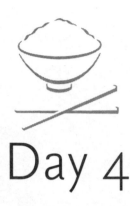

Day 4

Remember, the point of this plan is that it's psychological as well as nutritional. So today, as well as eating to fight stress, you should also think to fight it. A lot of us create stress in certain situations by imagining far worse outcomes than those that will actually occur. If you find yourself doing this today, instead, think: 'What's *really* going to happen?' It probably won't be nearly as bad as you fear.

Breakfast

2 slices malt loaf (about 2.5 cm/1 inch thick), topped with a little low-fat spread and 1 tablespoon low-sugar jam or honey. Serve with 200 ml (7 fl oz) skimmed milk. 2 small pieces of fruit such as plums or apricots.

Lunch

200 g (7 oz) any ready-made rice, pasta or couscous salad, topped with 1 tablespoon hummus and/or 2 slices turkey breast, served with cucumber slices.

Afternoon snack

4 oatcakes, topped with 1 teaspoon jam or honey.

Dinner

Seafood Quinoa Paella (see recipe on page 174), or top 50 g (2 oz) (dry weight) fettucine pasta with a simple sauce of unlimited sliced mushrooms, 200 g (7 oz) canned tomatoes, a little paprika and 1 tablespoon natural yogurt. Serve either of these with 2 slices of garlic bread and a small side salad.

Do the torch test

✲ Stress hormones are produced via the adrenal glands just above the kidneys. If you're under constant stress these can get fatigued – and so can you. To test if your adrenals are under pressure, shine a bright light onto your pupils while looking in a mirror. If they dilate, rather than contract, you need to adopt adrenal support tactics such as eating more high vitamin C foods and drinking licorice tea.

Seafood quinoa paella

1 teaspoon oil
15 g (½ oz) chorizo, chopped
1 clove garlic, chopped
1 small onion, chopped
1 chicken thigh, skinned and chopped
pinch of paprika
pinch of cayenne pepper
pinch of turmeric
2 medium tomatoes, chopped
75 g (3 oz) quinoa
250 ml (8 fl oz) stock
125 g (4 oz) cooked mixed seafood (such as squid, prawns, mussels)
1 tablespoon fresh parsley, chopped

Serves 1
Preparation time – 10 minutes
Cooking time – 45 minutes

Vegetarian option

✲ Replace the chorizo, chicken and seafood with 150 g canned pulses of your choice, drained and rinsed. Toss these through the paella before heating through and serving.

1 Heat the oil in a frying pan. Add the chorizo, garlic, onion and chicken and fry for 2 minutes.

2 Add all the remaining ingredients, except the seafood and parsley, and simmer for about 40 minutes until the quinoa is tender.

3 Add the seafood and parsley and heat through.

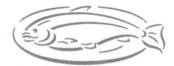

Day 5

Don't forget that one of the reasons stress leads to bloat is that we tend to bolt our meals when we're under pressure, increasing the amount of air we swallow. On this plan, therefore, take time over meals, chewing each mouthful 10–15 times. But also be aware of other factors that can increase the air you swallow, such as using sipper-style bottles, chewing gum and even having loose-fitting dentures.

Breakfast

40 g (1½ oz) bran cereal, topped with **150 ml (¼ pint) skimmed milk** and a **banana**. **3 oatcakes**, each topped with **1 teaspoon honey**.

Lunch

Open sandwich of **1 slice rye bread** spread with **25 g (1 oz) soft cheese**, topped with **75 g (3 oz) smoked salmon**, or **1 boiled egg**, served with a **salad** of **lettuce, cucumber, celery** and **green pepper**.

Afternoon snack

1 toasted crumpet, topped with **2 squares plain dark chocolate**, melted.

Dinner

125 g (4 oz) trout fillet, or **6 falafel balls**, grilled and served with **50 g (2 oz) (dry weight) couscous**, and **grilled red pepper slices**. Accompany with **1 tablespoon tzatsiki, hummus** or **salsa**.

Sleep your bloat away

✲ Stress is harder to handle if you're tired, so setting yourself a healthy sleep schedule that sees you getting 7–9 hours a night is going to help beat the bloat by calming you down. If you're a right-side sleeper, it might help you to switch to your left side. This stops any undigested food pressing on the opening of your oesophagus (which is on the right side of your stomach), which can cause indigestion and bloat.

Day 6

Today you may find that you get a sudden surge in energy. This is partly due to the regulation of your blood sugar levels, but if you're normally a coffee drinker it's also a sign that your symptoms of withdrawal, which take about four days to fade, are now over. Take note and remember that you can feel energized and motivated without using coffee as a crutch.

Breakfast

2 eggs, scrambled and mixed with 50 g (2 oz) smoked salmon or unlimited mushrooms and onion (both fried in a little oil spray). A handful of strawberries with 25 g (1 oz) feta cheese.

Lunch

2 slices granary bread, topped with 50 g (2 oz) sliced turkey or vegetarian bacon, ¼ avocado, sliced tomato and alfalfa sprouts. Serve with any 400 g (13 oz) can vegetable or lentil soup.

Afternoon snack

1 pear, apple or orange.

Dinner

125 g (4 oz) grilled gammon steak (fat removed), or ½ grilled aubergine, topped with 50 g (2 oz) cubed feta, chopped tomato and a handful of pumpkin seeds, served with 250 g (8 oz) sweet potato, mashed with a little yogurt and garlic, and unlimited broccoli.

Is alcohol making you stressed?

✣ While many of us have a drink to calm us when stressed, some people may actually be aggravated by alcohol. Research at the American National Institute of Mental Health found that some people suffer panic-attack symptoms as the effects of alcohol wear off – even after just one or two drinks. If you find yourself feeling more stressed the morning after drinking, maybe avoid it totally while on this plan.

Day 7

On this plan you're eating foods little and often, but try to eat your meals at the same times each day. Not only will this lead to more balanced levels of blood sugar, but research by Dr Ian MacDonald at the University of Nottingham, UK, has found that eating at set meal times increases metabolism and sees you burning 120 calories a day more than erratic eaters do.

Breakfast

Sandwich of **2 slices rye** or **granary bread** and **2 pork, turkey** or **vegetarian bacon rashers**, well grilled. Add a **little mustard** and some **sliced tomato**. **3–4 dried apricots** and a **handful** of **nuts** or **seeds**.

Lunch

1 large (50 g/2 oz) chicken or **vegetable samosa**, served with **1 teaspoon sweet chilli sauce**. Salad of **cucumber, tomato** and **onion** and **1 tablespoon tzatsiki**.

Afternoon snack

150 g (5 oz) pot low-fat custard with **2 handfuls of blueberries**.

Dinner

Beef and Sweet Potato Stew (see recipe on page 182), or any **350-calorie vegetarian ready meal** served with **unlimited green beans** and **50 g (2 oz) crusty French bread**.

Loosen your belt

✵ If you're feeling more het up than normal today, check your belt. As your stomach is shrinking, you may find you're feeling more confident with your slim shape and belting your waistbands more tightly. This constricts breathing, increasing levels of carbon dioxide in your system and boosting anxiety. Loosen things a notch, take some long slow breaths and see if you calm down.

Beef and sweet potato stew

125 g (4 oz) cubed stewing steak
seasoned flour to dust
2 teaspoons oil
1 carrot, chopped
1 small sweet potato, peeled and chopped
1 tablespoon tomato purée
250 ml (8 fl oz) good beef stock
1 tablespoon fresh herbs
   (such as rosemary, thyme, oregano), chopped

Serves 1
Preparation time – 10 minutes
Cooking time – about 1½ hours

Vegetarian option
❖ Replace the stewing steak with 125 g (4 oz) aubergine and replace the beef stock with vegetable stock.

1 Toss the beef in the seasoned flour.

2 Heat the oil in a medium-sized nonstick pan, add the beef and fry until browned all over.

3 Add the remaining ingredients, cover and simmer very gently for about 1¼ hours until the beef is tender.

4 Serve with steamed broccoli.

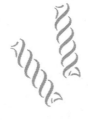

Day 8

Wherever you are today, take a few moments to reduce the amount of clutter around you. Piles of paper, children's toys and unpaid bills all gently increase the level of stress that you're under, meaning that it takes less to tip you over the edge. So spend ten minutes this morning filing, or at least removing clutter from the living room, to create a calmer environment in which to spend the day.

Breakfast

1 apple, cored and stuffed with 1 tablespoon mixed dried fruit. Bake at 200°C (400°F), Gas Mark 6, for 30 minutes, and serve with 125 g (4 oz) low-fat yogurt. 1 40 g (1½ oz) fruit scone, topped with 1 teaspoon low-sugar jam.

Lunch

200 g (7 oz) any ready-made pasta salad, served with unlimited green salad.

Afternoon snack

A handful of nuts and a banana.

Dinner

Quesadilla, made from 2 wholemeal tortillas filled with 50 g (2 oz) grated cheese and ¼ onion, fried. Microwave for 30 seconds to melt the cheese, top with salsa made from fresh chopped tomatoes with coriander, and serve with green salad.

Use your nose

✾ After you've cored today's breakfast apple, give it a sniff and inhale the aroma. Not only will this start your digestive processes working, helping to beat the bloat, but the scent of apple is also calming. Other stress-reducing odours include rosemary, vanilla and baked beans. Research at Middlesex University, UK, reveals the latter to be the number one food smell that makes people happy.

Day 9

By now, you may find you're getting fewer carb cravings than you used to suffer. This is partly because you're regulating your blood sugar levels and partly because you're supplying your brain with regular doses of serotonin. This means that your body no longer needs to send out distress signals when serotonin levels are low – signals that appear in the form of cravings for sugary or starchy foods.

Breakfast

2 wholewheat cereal 'biscuits', topped with 150 ml (¼ pint) warmed skimmed milk. Add 1 tablespoon raisins and 1 chopped apple and mix well. 1 slice wholemeal or granary toast topped with a little low-sugar jam.

Lunch

5 pieces sushi (such as **salmon, tuna, avocado, tofu**), served with **ginger, wasabi** and a cup of **miso soup**.

Afternoon snack

3 squares plain dark chocolate and 2 small pieces of fruit (such as **plums** or **apricots**).

Dinner

2 low-fat pork or **vegetarian sausages**, grilled and served with 250 g (8 oz) **sweet potato wedges** – cut sweet potato into large chunks, roast at 200°C (400°F), Gas Mark 6, for 20 minutes, shake, then roast for another 20 minutes – and **sliced leeks** and **onions**.

Slow and steady

✤ If you're still feeling het up, for seven minutes today try to breathe so slowly and steadily that you take just ten breaths over the space of a minute. Researchers at the University of Columbia, Missouri, USA, discovered that this is a very simple way to lower blood pressure and create a feeling of calm in the body. To get even more potent results, your in-breath should be roughly half as long as your out-breath.

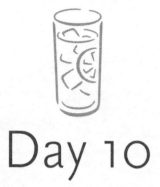

Day 10

We all know that stress makes us tired but,
if you're reducing stress yet still feel fatigued,
low iron levels could be to blame. To check yours,
look at your lower eyelid. If it's white or pale pink
(rather than red or dark pink), you are low in iron.
Adding a large serving of dark green vegetables
(such as spinach) to each meal or switching
to lean red meat instead of chicken
or fish can improve things.

Breakfast
2 small ready-made pancakes, topped with 1 teaspoon low-sugar jam. 200 ml (7 fl oz) fruit juice. 1 piece of fruit (such as orange, pear or banana) and a handful of nuts or seeds.

Lunch
4 oatcakes with 50 g (2 oz) low-fat, meat or vegetarian pâté. Add 6 pickled onions and unlimited celery sticks and cherry tomatoes.

Afternoon snack
150 g (5 oz) pot low-fat rice pudding.

Dinner
Root Vegetable Rösti-topped Fish Pie (see recipe on page 190), or any **350-calorie vegetarian ready meal** with 200 g (7 oz) mashed sweet potato. Serve either of these with unlimited green beans.

Recipe for calm
✲ If you haven't tried any of the recipes on this plan so far, then at least try today's – research shows that repetitive actions such as many of those used in cooking (kneading pastry, chopping vegetables or stirring, for example) are actually mini-meditations that calm your thoughts. Focusing on a recipe also stops you thinking about whatever is stressing you.

Root vegetable rösti-topped fish pie

125 g (4 oz) piece cod fillet, cubed
50 g (2 oz) prawns, defrosted if frozen
1 anchovy fillet
6 tablespoons light crème fraîche
1 tablespoon parmesan, grated
1 tablespoon fresh parsley, grated
1 small parsnip, parboiled
1 small potato, parboiled
1 teaspoon oil
freshly ground black pepper

Serves 1
Preparation time – 10 minutes
Cooking time – 30 minutes

Vegetarian option
✣ Replace the cod, prawns and anchovy fillet with chopped
Quorn pieces or a chopped Quorn fillet.

1 Preheat the oven to 200°C (400°F), Gas Mark 6.

2 Place the cod and prawns in a small ovenproof dish. Mash together the anchovy fillet, crème fraîche and parmesan. Stir through the parsley, season and pour over the fish.

3 Coarsely grate the parsnip, potato and carrot. Stir through the oil, then press the rösti onto the fish pie mixture.

4 Cook for 25–30 minutes until the topping is golden and the pie is bubbling.

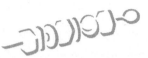

Day 11

Today's de-stress task is to do that one thing that's been nagging at you for ages – the phone call you've been putting off because it's unpleasant, or the expenses form you can't face filling in that's due next week. We don't consciously realize it, but loose ends such as this are always in the back of our mind and dealing with them can release massive amounts of tension.

Breakfast

2 slices rye or granary toast, topped with 250 g (8 oz) no-added-sugar baked beans. 2 cheese-spread triangles with 5–6 cherry tomatoes or grilled mushrooms.

Lunch

1 wholemeal bagel, topped with 1 pork, turkey or vegetarian bacon rasher and 2 slices of turkey and/or a boiled egg, plus a little mayonnaise and chopped lettuce and tomato. Serve with cucumber and carrot slices.

Afternoon snack

125 g (4 oz) low-fat yogurt, topped with 1 chopped apple.

Dinner

125 g (4 oz) prawns, or mozzarella cheese, made into kebabs with red peppers, onions and courgettes, grilled, served with 50 g (2 oz) (dry weight) rice and 2 tablespoons coleslaw.

Simple stress and bloat buster

✳ It's a packet of peppermints – not only does the herb mint calm the digestive system and help dissipate gas within the system, but studies from Jesuit University, West Virginia, USA, have found that the scent of peppermint helps decrease feelings of stress and frustration. Try popping a peppermint as a matter of course after meals to calm both your gut brain and your emotional one.

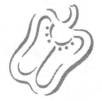

Day 12

If you find yourself wavering on the diet today, remind yourself that you're not just doing this to beat the bloat – you're also doing it to fight one of the most destructive things you can unleash on your system. The Chartered Institute of Personnel and Development, UK, says that stress accounts for six million sick days every year; by following this de-stress plan, you're lowering your risk of taking some of those sick days.

Breakfast

1 crumpet, topped with 1 teaspoon peanut butter and
1 sliced apple. A small punnet of blueberries.

Lunch

Open sandwiches of 2 slices thick rye bread, topped with
50 g (2 oz) low-fat feta cheese, roast red pepper slices and
a handful of olives. Serve with 400 g (13 oz) any lentil or
vegetable soup.

Afternoon snack

3–4 dried apricots and a handful of nuts or seeds.

Dinner

125 g (4 oz) chicken breast, halved and filled with 1 slice lean
ham and 25 g (1 oz) cheese, and then roast, or 1 large Portabella
mushroom, grilled and topped with 125 g (4 oz) tofu mixed with
1 teaspoon sweet chilli sauce. Serve either of these with 125 g
(4 oz) new potatoes and a large green salad.

De-stress your environment

✜ It's not just outside pressures that stress our system; factors
such as excess noise (even quiet, but irritating ones such as a
dripping tap), cold, heat or flickering lights can all increase our level
of arousal, making us feel minor stressors more acutely. During the
day today, do an audit of your surroundings and see what you need
to do to make yourself more comfortable.

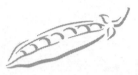

Day 13

If Day 13 falls at the weekend, make it a rule to do only the absolute essentials of chores, and then take the rest of the day off to have fun.

Most of us compound the stress of our working week by spending our weekends doing boring tasks, most of which (tidying the garage or washing the car, for example) aren't essential. Make it a new rule to keep at least one weekend day a month totally for you.

Breakfast
1 kipper, grilled, or 2 eggs, poached or scrambled, served with grilled tomatoes. 2 small pieces of fruit (such as satsumas, kiwifruit or apricots).

Lunch
Pitta pizza – spread a 65 g (2½ oz) pitta bread with a little tomato purée, top with 25 g (1 oz) grated cheese and unlimited vegetables (such as artichokes, olives, mushrooms), plus 5–6 anchovies if you eat them, then grill. Serve with a green salad, topped with a little balsamic vinegar.

Afternoon snack
3 squares plain dark chocolate and a handful of strawberries or raspberries.

Dinner
Gnocchi with Wild Mushroom and Spinach Sauce (see recipe on page 198), or a 350-calorie cottage/shepherd's pie ready meal. Serve either of these with unlimited peas.

Harness a childhood memory
✳ When you eat today's afternoon chocolate snack, don't chew it – suck it. We get calming sensations from sucking on something (one of the reasons why people turn to cigarettes when they're under pressure) as it reminds us of being fed as babies, which always made us feel good. Chocolate's a good food to try this with as it dissolves in heat – so after sucking for a short time you won't be swallowing large, unchewed particles.

Gnocchi with wild mushroom and spinach sauce

1 teaspoon oil
½ small onion, chopped
1 clove garlic, crushed
a few dried mushrooms, soaked in boiling water then drained and
   chopped
125 g (4 oz) fresh spinach
4 tablespoons light crème fraîche
1 tablespoon freshly grated parmesan
100 g (3½ oz) gnocchi, cooked according to packet instructions,
   drained
freshly ground black pepper

Serves 1
Preparation time – 10 minutes
Cooking time – 5 minutes

1 Heat the oil in nonstick frying pan. Add the onion and garlic and fry for 2 minutes.

2 Add the mushrooms and spinach and continue to fry for 2 minutes, until the spinach is wilted and any moisture has evaporated.

3 Stir in the crème fraîche, parmesan and the gnocchi and heat through. Season well.

Day 14

This is the last day of the diet and you should have noticed relief from both bloat and the amount of tension that you're under. But these might not be the only body boosts you're experiencing – stress affects so many areas of your physical being that you could find that your skin is clearer, you are suffering less back or neck pain, your headaches have vanished and even that your libido has increased.

Breakfast

1 small muffin (about 50 g/2 oz), served with 2 tablespoons blueberries and 125 g (4 oz) low-fat yogurt. 1 sliced pear and 25 g (1 oz) low-fat cheese.

Lunch

125 g (4 oz) turkey, or Quorn steak, served with 3 small roast potatoes, unlimited vegetables and 1–2 tablespoons gravy.

Afternoon snack

3 oatcakes, topped with honey or jam.

Dinner

1 wholemeal tortilla spread with a little harissa paste or salsa, and 1 tablespoon tzatsiki. Fill with 125 g (4 oz) sliced lamb, chicken or ½ avocado and grated carrot and onion. Serve with a side salad.

Do you have a secret stressor?

✣ If, even after all your efforts of the last fortnight, you still feel stressed but aren't sure why, try this test. Hold out your arm and ask a friend to push down on it as you resist. While they do this, think of things going on in your life. When you reach the thing that's really stressing you, your arm will go weak and you won't be able to resist the pressure. Once you know your secret stressor, it will be easier to tackle it.

What to do when the diet is over

By now, you should be feeling significantly calmer and more in control of your life and your body, and have probably sworn to avoid stressful situations for ever – but that isn't good for you either. Short bursts of pressure (such as 1–2 days under a deadline) not only motivate us to get things done, but research shows that they also increase levels in the body of a hormone called DHEA-S that boosts libido and memory and lowers weight. The key, though, is switching off from the stress when it's done (or at least when you leave the workplace) and here are six ways you can do just that.

1 Follow the 3:1 ratio. As explained, carbohydrate foods help your body to produce the calming hormone serotonin and, while eating them alone gives the fastest response, your body also needs protein to stay well. Therefore, according to leading nutrition researcher Dr Pamela Peeke from the University of Maryland, USA, the ideal ratio for long-term stress control and good health is 75 g (3 oz) of carbohydrate (both starchy and fruit and vegetables) for every 25 g (1 oz) of protein on your plate per meal.

2 Increase your vitamin C levels when you know you're going to be under pressure. Studies at the University of Trier, Germany, found that when levels of vitamin C in the body are high we have lower blood pressure and lower cortisol levels and feel less stressed by pressures than when they are low. Foods high in vitamin C include blueberries, red peppers, kiwifruit, citrus fruit and potatoes.

3 Don't be afraid of healthy fats. While saturated fat seems to increase levels of stress hormones, there's a lot of evidence showing that healthy omega-3 fats reduce the impact of stress on the body. Make sure your diet includes nuts, seeds, oily fish, olives, avocado – or healthy oils such as flaxseed to help bolster your body's defences.

4 Harness natural helpers. There are many of these that can fight stress – from '*avena sativa*' (derived from oats; see page 163), which creates calming sensations in your body, to aromatherapy oils, such as lavender, that produce calming alpha waves in your brain. Particularly helpful are Bach flower remedies, which aim to act on specific thoughts and feelings that cause stress – for example, centuary helps you fight the fear of saying no, while elm helps you tackle feelings of responsibility. You'll find all of these at health stores.

5 If your stomach reacts to stress, take a probiotic supplement. It seems that there's nothing in our body that having low levels of these healthy gut bacteria doesn't influence – and the reaction of our body to stress is one of them. Studies at McMaster University, Canada, have found that high levels of good gut bacteria reduce muscle spasms of the gut during stress, meaning you'll suffer less digestive discomfort, including cramps and bloat.

6 Build some exercise into each day. It will lower the levels of stress hormones in your body and therefore reduce the effects they can have on you. Aerobic exercise helps burn off chemicals that make you jittery (even a ten-minute walk will have some effects), but gentler, yet cerebral exercise such as yoga or tai chi helps lower stress levels by relaxing your mind. In fact, studies show that even your very first session of yoga can dramatically lower cortisol levels – imagine how calm you'll be if you do it regularly.

Index

Acknowledgements

Executive Editor Nicky Hill
Editor Lisa John
Design Manager Tokiko Morishima
Designer Barbara Zuñiga
Production Manager Ian Paton

Author Acknowledgements
Thanks to the various experts I've interviewed in the past who have helped me acrue the knowledge to write this book – particularly Natalie Savona, Neil Wooten, Dr John Mansfield and Patrick Holford. And to Tim, who, yet again, supplied the tea and wine required to get to deadline day.